The *Animal* HEALER

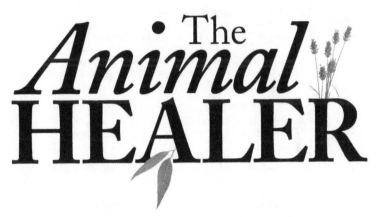

•The
Animal
HEALER

A Unique Insight into the Healing,
Care and Wellbeing of Animals

Elizabeth Whiter
with Gilly Smith

HAY HOUSE

Australia • Canada • Hong Kong • India
South Africa • United Kingdom • United States

First published and distributed in the United Kingdom by:
Hay House UK Ltd, 292B Kensal Rd, London W10 5BE. Tel.: (44) 20 8962 1230;
Fax: (44) 20 8962 1239. www.hayhouse.co.uk

Published and distributed in the United States of America by:
Hay House, Inc., PO Box 5100, Carlsbad, CA 92018-5100. Tel.: (1) 760 431 7695 or
(800) 654 5126; Fax: (1) 760 431 6948 or (800) 650 5115. www.hayhouse.com

Published and distributed in Australia by:
Hay House Australia Ltd, 18/36 Ralph St, Alexandria NSW 2015. Tel.: (61) 2 9669 4299;
Fax: (61) 2 9669 4144. www.hayhouse.com.au

Published and distributed in the Republic of South Africa by:
Hay House SA (Pty), Ltd, PO Box 990, Witkoppen 2068. Tel./Fax: (27) 11 467 8904.
www.hayhouse.co.za

Published and distributed in India by:
Hay House Publishers India, Muskaan Complex, Plot No.3, B-2, Vasant Kunj,
New Delhi – 110 070. Tel.: (91) 11 4176 1620; Fax: (91) 11 4176 1630. www.hayhouse.co.in

Distributed in Canada by:
Raincoast, 9050 Shaughnessy St, Vancouver, BC V6P 6E5. Tel.: (1) 604 323 7100;
Fax: (1) 604 323 2600

A catalogue record for this book is available from the British Library.

ISBN 978-1-84850-190-4

Spike photo: Courtesy of Mia Sampietro
Merlin photo: Courtesy of Porcupine PR
Celia Hammond Cat Trust photo: Courtesy of Lisa Moss

Disclaimer: Spiritual healing is *not* a substitute for professional veterinary care. Hands-on
healing is complementary, and a great support to any veterinary care, but if you are in any
doubt about the welfare of your animal(s), a vet must always be your first port of call.

Once in a lifetime someone truly amazing comes along, like Elizabeth Whiter. Without Elizabeth we would be without our dog Frosty. There is no doubt that her healing powers, herbal remedies and dietary advice have worked a miracle in keeping Frosty alive and well against the odds.

SHAUN AND CHRISTINE

Elizabeth Whiter's energy and enthusiasm for her work is quickly transferred to the animals in her care, with wonderful results. The animals in our care have benefited from her expertise in healing, work with oils and great compassion.

SIOBHAN LORD, EQUINE MARKET WATCH SANCTUARIES

When the vet said that the best thing might be to put our dog Woody to sleep, my family were devastated. Elizabeth sent remote healing to Woody, and within a short time his energy had changed, he was brighter and the spark was back in his eye. Elizabeth has given me hope, hope that there are good human beings out there who devote their lives to our animal friends and ask nothing back. I'm sincerely grateful.

SALLY

We have been working with Liz for many years now with great results for a wide variety of our animals and birds including our wildlife casualties. Liz has had an amazing impact on our resident barn owl, Merlin, and on our boa constrictor, Sidney, who are completely relaxed in her presence. The techniques we have learned through her workshops and courses help our animals every day and we have achieved good success rates in rehabilitating the garden birds, hedgehogs, bats and birds of prey who come into our care.

STEVE SHORE, THE ACORN PROJECT

Meeting Liz and attending her courses has changed my life for ever by opening up a whole new world of opportunity, and enabling me to make fantastic new friendships! Thank you, Liz, keep up the good work.

Hazel

Liz bounced into our shelter with energy enough to make everyone smile and immediately respond to her natural enthusiasm and talent for loving and understanding humans and animals alike. It's no wonder animals respond so readily to her methods of healing.

Sharon, Nicosia Dog Shelter

Dedicated to all my sisters and brothers in the animal kingdom. This book is for you.

Acknowledgements

First and foremost, my thanks goes to my husband Brian
for supporting my vision and encouraging me to realise the
dream, and for feeding our menagerie of animals day and
night while I spent endless days, nights and months tapping
away on the computer. I kept hearing your voice in my head
saying, 'It's team work, baby.' It sure is! You are my anchor,
you are my life and I love you.

Enormous gratitude and love to Gilly, my dear friend,
colleague and mentor, who has helped me make this dream
project come true, providing professional and personal
support throughout the whole of this incredible two-year
writing process.

To my best friends – my mum and my sister Susie – who
have supported me every step of the way on my healing
journey.

In loving memory of my dad, who was my hero and gave
me solid roots from which to grow and flourish.

Heartfelt thanks and appreciation to Michelle Pilley at Hay
House, who has been a guiding light and inspiration to me.
I thank everybody at Hay House UK – a dynamic
publishing house with great team spirit and dedication.
Special thanks to Leanne Siu Anastasi for the design of

this book, and many thanks to Joanna Lincoln, Amanda Wheeler, Jo Burgess, Louise Firth, Amy Kiberd and Barbara Vesey.

Grateful thanks to Lee, Peter and Anita at Magik Thread for believing in me and encouraging me to write this book.

Special thanks to Holly, Mia, Maddie, Diane, Sue, Tracey, Alison, Vanessa, Amanda, Helen and Robbie for supporting me while I was creating the manuscript, teaching the diploma in animal healing and working at the animal healing clinic.

Thanks to all of my hard-working students and graduates who have become great friends and healing colleagues.

To other friends I may have failed to mention here by name, but love to you all unconditionally

Many thanks to Lee, my gifted web designer, technical advisor and computer whizz!

Special thanks to all the veterinarians, animal care and rescue workers, animal guardians and vet nurses I have had the privilege of working with and the incredible work you do with animals.

Contents

Part Five: What We Know Now

Part Six: Recipes

Foreword

When Elizabeth Whiter asked me to write a foreword for her new book, I was busy treating her horse Betty for a severe suspensory ligament injury. The hind limb was very swollen around the hock, and initially a hock injury was feared. A closer inspection identified that the fetlock of the affected limb was lower than the other hind fetlock, and I suspected an injury of the suspensory ligament. An ultrasound examination confirmed this diagnosis and a treatment plan was formulated. The mare also had a foal at foot which needed to be weaned as well, complicating matters. During this process Elizabeth asked me what she herself could do to help Betty as well, and she suggested several treatments that would be supportive. Among these were a seaweed wrap placed underneath the support bandage and self-selected garlic. With the aid of conventional veterinary medicine and Elizabeth's knowledge of healing (as well as good old TLC!) we managed to reduce the swelling and heat and make the mare more comfortable.

The first time I met Elizabeth was several years ago when I had to examine one of her other horses. At the end of that first visit Elizabeth introduced me to the world of herbs and oils. Sparkling with energy, she showed me around her herb garden and had me taste rose hips and other herbal products. We had an interesting discussion about complementary medicine, and I, being a very factual person used to evidence that is backed up by peer-reviewed science, remember being quite sceptical at first. But I was very impressed by Elizabeth's extensive knowledge of natural remedies. This was combined with a sound approach towards the emotional relationship that exists between pet owners and their animals.

I am no stranger to complementary medicine as I have recently used medical-grade maggots to remove necrotic tissue from delicate and deep wounds that are infected with antibiotic-resistant bacteria. This is a treatment dating back to ancient times, but went out of fashion with the discovery of penicillin. However, modern medicine is now forced to look for alternative treatments with the rise of so-called 'superbugs'. And I do believe that there are many herbs and plants out there that may have medicinal properties that we do not know of, yet. People like Elizabeth Whiter may help us teach and understand this knowledge, which has been collected over thousands of years.

Let there be no mistaking the fact that modern technologies have enabled veterinary medicine to make an accurate diagnosis, and have earned their place. The fact that many injuries are cared for with a plethora of different treatments means only that there is no perfect one. It may well be that, in cases such as these, complementary healing can make a valuable contribution to a solution.

Egbert M O Willems
DVM CertES(Orth) MRCVS

Introduction

I sit here in my kitchen in the heart of a Sussex summer, with the sun blazing outside as I crush some fresh aloe vera from a plant on the window-sill and my young Norfolk terriers Lily and Morris snooze at my feet. Lovely old Alf, my 14-year-old long-haired Jack Russell, is pottering about in the garden, and our black cat Tao (whom we've nicknamed Mrs T) is sitting on the gate keeping her huge green eyes on everything around her. I feel truly blessed.

It's hard to believe that my old boss at the *Daily Mail* once bought me a fold-up bed because I was spending so much time in the office. Back in the eighties, I was an ambitious hard-working professional woman, the youngest person at the *Mail* and dead set on making my mark. By the time I'd launched one of the first property sections to appear in a national newspaper, I was the golden girl – but I had no life to speak of at all. I was living in the heart of London but felt like the loneliest girl on the planet. Pretty soon I was burnt out, lonely, confused about what job satisfaction really meant to me, and ready for a change.

A career in sales for a pharmaceutical publisher, setting up deals across Europe, earned me the cash for a lifestyle change. For a while, to support my new show jumper husband Nat, I juggled the huge financial implications of keeping the show on the road. Before long, though, I was sacrificing a precious home life for gruelling hours and lonely hotels in an attempt to pay for the upkeep of our horses and the expense of the shows. I yearned to be around the horses with Nat, but as the sole breadwinner I was struggling to pay the mortgage each month. I felt I was on a treadmill going nowhere. I was never at home. And when Nat left me for a younger woman after only two years of marriage, I realized I hadn't even noticed the cracks that had been gaping in my life plan for a good while.

It was my animals who gave me the opportunity to live the life I really wanted to lead, and who showed me that there are choices everywhere. Now, I spend my days working with animals who do the same for *their* owners.

I will be honest with you: the transition from one life to another was painful. I took Nat's betrayal terribly personally and my self-esteem was on the floor. But today I am thankful, because I learned so much from what turned out to be one of my most valuable life experiences. At the time it appeared to be the end of the world, but pulling myself from the darkest depths and rising up to where I am now was a truly cathartic experience.

I had the choice to stay a victim and drown in my sorrows and repeat the same life patterns or to dust myself down and start again. I chose the latter. After a period of grieving and re-evaluating what I wanted from my life, I realized that I didn't have to sell my soul to pay the mortgage and I began to feel strong enough to think about what I really wanted from my life.

So many people rush into relationships, but I knew that I had to take the time to recover from Nat before I could move into a healthy relationship. For me now, having recognized that there is so much synchronicity in my life, it's no surprise that Brian came along when I was ready – but at the time it seemed like a miracle. He has been my rock now for the last 13 years, and has always allowed me the space to develop into who I really am. While I was supporting Nat, I had felt like a racehorse with blinkers on, intent only on what was in front of me. Meeting Brian lit up a whole new space to think.

Our honeymoon period was cut short, however, one balmy autumn evening in 1996. My horse Wow, a nine-year-old Danish-bred grey gelding show jumper, was involved in a horrific accident that night, and the events that would follow would push me almost over the edge with grief.

I had decided to leave Wow out instead of bringing him in for the night, and he was rugged up in a secure paddock next to the house. In the middle of the night, a freak autumn storm rose up and, terrified, Wow jumped the five-foot gate, all 16.3 hands of him, galloped down the grassy lane and fell into a neighbour's swimming pool. The pool was full of water with a canvas covering, and Wow had to fight for his life, laden down with the weight of his own rug which was saturated in water. Somehow he found the strength to scramble out of the pool and make his way back to his field.

When I found him the next morning, his legs and throat were cut and bruised, yet when the vet came to see him, after a thorough examination he simply treated Wow for shock. Wow had trotted up sound and none of us detected that his state was more serious than it appeared.

Over the next six months Wow continued to deteriorate, yet veterinary specialists still could not find the problem. Determined to find the answer, I took him to the Animal Health Trust near Cambridge for a scintigraphy scan – an injection of a purple dye that reveals 'hot spots' where there has been damage to the vertebrae. The vet confirmed that Wow had broken his neck in three places. The prognosis was not good and the vet recommended that we put him down.

Devastated, I boxed Wow up and drove home, weeping all the way. I felt so useless, angry and powerless. Why Wow? He was the most kind-hearted, lovable horse I had ever known. He was such a gentleman.

That evening as I sat with him in his stable, something strange began to happen. I could sense just how emotionally drained and depressed he was, and I felt compelled to stand up and slowly walk around him, stroking him gently and putting my hands close to various parts of his broken body.

Instinctively I was drawn to the areas of his body that needed my touch. I felt incredibly relaxed yet my attention was solely on Wow. My body even felt different; I seemed to have grown. My feet were like magnets, pulling me into the ground, and I felt a sense of calmness and strength throughout the whole of my body. A wave of happiness swept over me, a feeling of total euphoria.

I noticed that Wow was breathing to my rhythm; it was as if we were synchronized. It was an extraordinary, harmonious moment. A silence enveloped the stable and a feeling far greater than happiness swept over my body. It was a stillness, a purity. It took me back to the feeling that I had had when I saw Robert Powell's TV portrayal of Christ in *Jesus of Nazareth*. Like then, this feeling was almost an epiphany, something incredibly powerful that was to change my life.

Wow seemed to be getting comfort from me and, as I whispered to him, he began to relax and sigh. I had never done anything like this before with him. It just felt right. I knew nothing about healing – in fact, at that time, I didn't even know what the term meant – but I loved my horse so much that I couldn't bear the thought of having to put him down. I would have done anything to help him.

After that evening, I spent more and more time with him. After a good day's grazing in the field, Wow liked to retire to his stable at night. While he was munching his hay, I would lean over the stable door and see if it was a good time. He always ushered me in by gently nudging my arm and shoulders. As I put my hands close to him, he would swing his head round and guide me to areas he wanted me to work on, and very gradually I began to sense for myself where to put my hands, feeling different sensations in my palms. Sometimes they became hot, while other places made them cold, tingly or throbbing, with a low-frequency hum that seemed to be vibrating from my palms.

I watched Wow's reactions carefully; he would sigh and go into a deeply relaxed state, sometimes nodding off, resting a back leg and allowing his head and neck to drop slightly and relax even further. Sometimes 20 minutes would pass without my noticing. At other times, it would feel right to stop. Sometimes Wow would walk away, but at the end of a session he always looked me in the eye and I felt he was thanking me.

It felt remarkable to have this kind of communication with my beloved horse. It seemed that both of us were being healed. But I didn't believe that Wow was going to get better just by my putting his hands near him. I knew now that his neck had been badly broken and even though his spirit seemed stronger after our sessions together, he needed more than my hands if he was going to recover.

That summer following Wow's accident, Brian and I moved our two horses, Wow and our beautiful brown mare, Betty, as well as Alf the Jack Russell and Bruce the boxer, to our new home in Sussex. We were in the middle of unpacking when Betty snagged her head on barbed wire and needed a stitch. Andrew Browning, my new equine vet, came to treat her and, as I introduced him to Wow, I suddenly found myself bursting into tears and telling him the story. I'm sure that the emotional upheaval of the move was responsible for such an uncharacteristic outburst, but he was very kind and listened to the whole tale. He reassuringly put his arm around me and told me about a new technique he was working on with Anthony Pusey, a respected osteopath whose ground-breaking work was rippling through the equine world. He was gaining a highly credible reputation after treating the Queen's horses. He asked me to bring Wow to his clinic the following week, and a wave of relief swept over me. This was the first time anyone had ever given me any hope for Wow.

First, though, I needed to set to work on the mammoth task of making our rambling old house and land into a home. I was wondering how on earth I was going to deal with the fencing, the poo-picking, the painting and decorating of a house that had been in a time warp for years, when a friend called by to ask how I was getting on. I told her how overwhelmed I felt at the prospect of so much work and asked if she knew anyone who might be able to help. She worked at a local tea shop in the heart of the community, and suggested that I give her my number so that she could pass it on if she heard of anyone looking for extra work. I thanked her and started planning my trip with Wow to the clinic.

The night before the trip to the osteopath, I went into Wow's stable and again I felt an overwhelming desire to place my hands near his neck and pelvis. Wow had now become used to these daily sessions and was perfectly happy to let me learn with him. Despite the advice from most of the experts, I didn't feel pessimistic about Wow any more. I felt powerful and positive about wanting to make him better. It was a feeling of joy and unconditional love.

I arrived early at the clinic and settled Wow into his stable before going to get a coffee. As I was waiting for the kettle to boil, I started chatting to another client who had brought her horse to see Tony Pusey. We exchanged names and she seemed startled when she heard mine. 'Elizabeth Whiter?' she repeated. 'I've heard of you.' I told her that I had only recently moved to the area, but she was already rummaging in her bag and pulling out a crumpled piece of paper with my name on. 'That's my writing,' I said, astonished. She told me that she had been given it in a tea room a couple of days before by the lady who worked there. She had been chatting to a friend about wanting to work with horses again, and the tea lady (while apologizing for eavesdropping) had handed my details to her.

Although Vanessa had a business of her own to run, we chatted about the possibility of her helping me out, and she told me about the healing centre she ran in the city. I was so excited by the synchronicity of what was happening, and by having met someone who might be able to understand what I had been experiencing with Wow, that I began to tell her about it. 'You were healing him!' she laughed as I tried to find the words to describe what I had been doing. 'I think you should come and visit the centre. We've got lots of self-development courses and workshops you might be interested in.' I felt as if I had come home.

It was time for Wow's appointment. I watched in amazement as Tony Pusey strapped himself into a body protector and got to work. He looked like the Michelin Man as he waddled towards Wow's stable. He spent about half an hour manipulating Wow's whole spine and quickly confirmed that Wow had suffered three really bad breaks and was lucky to be alive. He said he had never seen anything as bad as this, and that he could not believe how composed and calm Wow was.

I explained what I had been doing in Wow's stable, and he told me that he had used a local anaesthetic to induce a similar state of deep relaxation to enable him to manipulate Wow's bones. He told me that he believed that the preparation I had done the night before meant that he hadn't had to use as much anaesthetic with Wow as he would expect to use on a new patient.

Wow went on to have treatments with Tony Pusey for the next year. There was no question in my mind about following this through to completion, but Tony told me that many of his clients would start a course of treatment for their horses but then give up soon afterwards. I know now that commitment is one of the most important factors in successful healing.

I learned so much from those sessions. Vanessa had given me a new word to describe what I was trying to achieve, and it seemed like my whole world was opening up because of Wow's accident. My address book was filling with a new team of exciting people who were helping me to see all my animals in a completely different way, and I was fascinated by every new piece of the jigsaw that each of these complementary therapists was showing me. I drank up as much information as I could get.

Twelve years on I am, as far as I know, one of the only people in the UK with a clinic which heals both pets *and* their owners. I'm a qualified complementary therapist in healing, nutrition, kinesiology and zoopharmacognosy, and a member of The Ingraham Institute of Zoopharmacognosy.

I teach a diploma course in animal healing with 30 students passing through my 'school' every year who learn almost everything that I have learned, from bereavement counselling to anatomy and physiology, so that this therapy can truly complement the work of other animal professionals. It is a vital part of the courses I offer that students gain a solid grounding in all aspects of animal healing – physical, emotional and spiritual.

Much of the work that I did in my training and since has resulted in strong links and relationships with vets, dog trainers and animal behaviourists, and although there is no typical day at the clinic, it's very likely that I will start my day with a referral from one of these fellow professionals. I do get phone calls from people who want to bypass the vet and bring their animals straight to me, but I tell them that they must get a diagnosis from their vet first.

I like to think of us all working together as a hub. I have some animals who are terminally ill and others with behaviour problems. I might see a dog with an old injury sustained years before and which is now developing into arthritis, and others with congenital issues such as heart problems or epilepsy. Their owners may be working with other experts and come in for just a couple of sessions, but they often refer to all of us as their 'team'. I love that. Animals are living so much longer now and they need support for the kind of elderly conditions that any of us will suffer from. This is where complementary therapies can really help; a bit of time and understanding can work wonders when a dog is becoming deaf or slowing down. Owners often worry about whether or not they are doing the best for their ageing animal; spending time supporting their pet can really help them make good decisions.

Watching animals select the plants (and the oils extracted from these plants) that their ancestors would have naturally foraged in order to heal themselves in the wild was one of the most humbling parts of the diploma course I put myself through. Recognizing just how in touch animals are with what they need rearranged my ideas of the master and servant relationship for ever!

But it was the moment when Wow showed himself to be the beautiful, communicative, receptive soul that he is, that changed my life. It's something I witness in pet owners and their animals most days in my own clinic now, especially as the animals so often mirror their owners' needs. The terrier's skin conditions, the cat's cancer, the mare's aggression are, in part, outward indications of things not being right at home. I never get tired of witnessing the transformation as the owner sees just how connected his pet is to him and vice versa. It makes me wonder how I ever lived without the communication I now have with my animals.

Our pets' unconditional love for us, and their deep understanding of what we need in our own lives, has given me another kind of drive, a greater ambition than I ever had at the *Mail* or the publishing company. For me, the power to heal is about the power to communicate what it is that animals and their owners need; to tell the world that the universal capacity for love, connection and communication can be the biggest healer of them all.

And Wow? Would you believe that he was even able to jump again for one final season? Today, at 21 years old, he is leading a full and stimulating life, hacking out every week across the Sussex countryside, lending a wise old ear to my young horse, Dancer, and our new foal, Iris, and helping to rehabilitate a beautiful young girl with epilepsy. He is my best example when I am giving healing lectures and workshops. He has a Buddha energy that comes from really understanding what suffering is and how to learn from it. He is my greatest teacher and friend, and I dedicate this book to him.

PART ONE
The Journey Home

The soul is the same in all living creatures,
although the body of each is different.
HIPPOCRATES

Learning to Meditate

No two days are the same for me in the clinic. I might see three or four animal patients and their owners in the course of a day, or I might be out visiting horses in a nearby yard. I might be lecturing on animal husbandry at an agricultural college, or working at the bat hospital. I could be in a rescue centre 50 miles away, or getting ready to travel to a rescue centre abroad where my healing skills are needed for the many abandoned animals who find their way there.

I've come down a long path since I first found myself putting my hands close to Wow, a practice which I have since learned is part of spiritual healing or prayer work and which is recognized by the Royal College of Veterinary Surgeons.

I have learned an entirely new set of skills over the last ten years, and I've been completely committed to the incredible training that is so important for this work since the day I discovered that I had the ability to heal.

Professional development can never be achieved overnight and, unlike many other healing courses, it takes much longer than a weekend. The courses that I have been on and the people I have met have literally changed my life, and when I open my clinic in the mornings I never fail to thank God for this extraordinary place where I am now.

After meeting Vanessa and beginning the meditation classes with her, I found that I was driven by a new energy, a thirst for knowledge that had come from my new-found ability to heal. I remember that moment when the vet said that there was nothing more that I could do for Wow: an incredibly powerful feeling awoke inside me. I would not let my horse die. It was the spark that set the healer in me alight and I was ready to do anything I could to help him, to jump into a totally new world full of opportunities.

I have always been interested in working with animals. As a little girl, I dreamed of being a vet when I grew up, but, although I loved biology at school, as much as I tried I just couldn't get to grips with chemistry and physics, which I needed in order to train as a vet, and so my life took a different path. Sometimes I have to pinch myself now to realize that my dream actually did come true, although not in the way that I thought it would. I had no idea that I would be working with animals myself as an intuitive animal healer.

After I found that my hands were pulsating when I put them around Wow, I learned that the laying on of hands is an age-old instrument in the healer's tool box. The more I talked to people in the complementary health world, the wider my knowledge about healing became, and the more committed I was to improving my understanding of it.

I have learned that it is important to meditate before a healing in order to ground myself and to expand my energy. When I was first learning to meditate, however, I found it hard to focus. It was so easy to allow my mind to drift off. I remembered that Vanessa had told me about a meditation group at a local complementary health centre which held guided meditations. I decided to try it to see if I could focus better with the help of others around me.

I loved it. The energy in the room was blissful after a session, and it was so lovely to see all those peaceful, smiling eyes after a guided meditation. I really felt that I was transported in those sessions, and I felt encouraged to try to get that focus in my own meditations at home.

I noticed that my healings were becoming more powerful as my mind learned to become still. By this time I had only healed Wow, but I started putting my hands close to Betty, my mare, and Alf, my dog. I knew now how to attune myself first, grounding my energy into the earth, breathing and focusing my attention on the animals. I was amazed at the response. Alf rolled over almost immediately, sighing with contentment, and then seemed to direct me to different parts of his body, exposing his stomach at one point and moving his back end to me at another as if to say, 'Here, please.'

I had always thought I had communicated quite naturally with my animals. Like most owners, I had always chatted, stroked and praised them without thinking twice about it.

But this was different. I noticed for the first time that my animals would let me know where they needed attention. The more I understood their body language, and they mine, the more time we wanted to spend with each other. All these years on, I have radically transformed my relationships with my animals. When my mare Betty was pregnant with little Iris, our healing sessions brought all three of us so much closer to each other. In the stable Betty seemed to be actively seeking healing; she seemed to know the benefits for herself, and wanted the same for her rapidly growing foetus. She would push her expanding belly into my hands, and when she wanted further healing elsewhere, she would rest a near back leg, so I could reach up and heal her pelvis, as if to say, 'This is where I need it.' It felt such a privilege; I could feel the trust Betty gave me as the healing energy reached out to baby Iris in the womb. I could see the little movements as her weight drew closer to the side I was healing. The birth was easy and relaxed, and Iris is already a happy, confident little foal.

I know now that healing is a conscious intention, while casual cuddles are an automatic expression of love. Stroking a cat can help its owner zone out and relax, but healing comes from deliberately altering your state of mind. Meditation is an essential part of this.

The power of meditation as part of the healing process is now well understood and has been embraced by the National Health Service as a welcome and effective contribution to cancer care. It is a fundamental part of my healing sessions and, after a consultation, I always invite the client to join me in a meditation so that we can create a quiet space in our minds and access the stillness in us and around the pet patient.

I encourage them to take the practice home with them and try it out in their own time, but many of them tell me they are worried that they're not 'doing it right'. Of course there is a procedure, a way of focusing that can help, but once the intention is there to calm the mind, and to send love out into the world, you simply can't do anything wrong. It can be hard to calm a busy brain, but I find that the more that meditation becomes part of your daily routine, the easier it is to switch off.

Some people like to sit outside for their practice, particularly in the early morning when the natural world is beginning to wake up, or at dusk when everything is settling down again after a busy day. After living in London for six years, just being in the countryside can bring on the feeling of blissful peace that meditation can inspire. I can barely leave the countryside now without getting withdrawal symptoms.

I know plenty of people who can meditate perfectly easily in their bedroom or, if there's no one around, on the sitting room floor, but I choose to meditate in a room specifically laid out for the purpose. I have a set time when I turn off the phones and tell everyone who needs to know that I'm not available. The room is very beautiful and gently lit by candlelight, with cushions scattered on the floor where I can comfortably sit for the next hour.

The act of focusing on a special place tends to stop the mind drifting off. Most people are visual and can quite easily imagine a beautiful place like a lake, a meadow or a place that they loved as a child. For those who find sounds more soothing, a tape or CD can really help to guide a meditation.

My favourite place to focus on is a forest glade with a shaft of light shining through the trees. I can feel the warmth on my skin almost immediately, and it seems that I really am right there. My feet become rooted into the ground as I imagine that I am a very old tree, planted deeply into the ancient earth with my leaves reaching for the sunlight. Once I feel connected to the earth and to the universal energy all around me, I can begin to quieten my mind.

Meditation is about more than just finding a bit of peace and quiet after a busy day. It's about feeling part of the universe, connecting with something bigger than us. One of the most common issues I come across among my human clients is the feeling of being alone, unconnected. The simple act of meditation, sitting down and tapping into the earth's energy under the feet, can root us, reminding us of the millions of years' worth of experience and activity which gives us a sense of context and meaning to our lives. Meditation grounds us. It's when the ego takes a break from looking after number one and remembers the bigger picture.

I have witnessed Liz blossom while sacrificing her old life, and never giving up on her dreams. 'Life is a journey, not a destination' was never more apt than when attributed to Liz. She has boundless energy, enthusiasm and love for the world and all who inhabit it.
VANESSA, ONE-TIME OWNER OF THE HOLISTIC HEALTH CENTRE

The Healing Meditation

Grounding exercises ensure that I am protected from any external influences such as grief or anxiety, and help me stay focused and positive. Without proper grounding, anyone could easily find themselves giving away their own energy reserves; after a busy day at the clinic, my energy would pretty soon become depleted.

The tree analogy that I use in my personal meditation works very well in the grounding exercise. Most people can easily visualize the roots of a tree sinking heavily through their feet and extending way down into the earth, and the leaves absorbing all that natural sun energy as they reach out and up to the sky. If I'm working with a client who is new to meditation, I use a breathing exercise, focusing on breathing in and expanding the diaphragm and then letting the breath empty from the lungs to help to calm the mind, release any tension and restore the most wonderful sense of peace.

The grounding exercise is an essential tool in switching the power of thought to the positive, and the relief it gives can be very profound. There are often a lot of tears in my clinic as clients realize just how negative their own self-belief is. Very often a dog will come over and lick his companion, but it feels more of an empathetic lick than a sympathetic one. Scientists have discovered that 'mirror neurons' – the specific nerve cells associated with empathy, the bedrock of social emotions – physically exist in the brain of humans, some primates, birds and maybe even other mammals. I see evidence of this almost every day.

Once we are relaxed, I ask both of us to concentrate on sending loving thoughts to the animal patient, as I gently place my hands around his body. Apart from a gentle stroke, I rarely touch the animal and am aware that there will be sensitive areas which he will not want me to approach. I always keep my eyes open so I can monitor his responses and facial expressions. My hands will be pulsating with energy by now and as I feel the hot and cold spots in various parts of the body, I direct that energy to the neediest areas. The animal will often guide me to the areas of pain by getting up and moving a back leg nearer to my hands or putting his nose to the area needing attention. It's a lovely moment for the client to watch a pet asking for and getting what he needs.

I like us to remain in silence while I am healing animals so I can completely focus, leaving the chat to the end, but the animal may get up and move around or even away from me. Whatever happens is fine; the animal usually comes back for some more healing pretty quickly as the focus is so intensely on him and most beings can't resist that. When one of my new clients, Suzanna, first brought her cat Suki down from London with a problem with her breathing, she explained that Suki was a very fearful cat and really only responded to her. She was amazed when Suki edged out of her cat basket and sat quietly while I placed my hands around her. After a quarter of an hour, Suki was butting me with her head in a way that Suzanna had never seen her do with strangers before. Pouring that amount of love into an animal will always have a wonderful effect, but when the energy in the room is filled with peace and calm, animals just can't get enough. Once Suki was relaxed and open, she was able to absorb the healing more effectively, and Suzanna basked in it, too.

It's vital for both of us to 'close down' at the end of a healing meditation, to draw the energy back into the body, breathing out any anxieties or negative thoughts, and breathing in and filling up with a bigger, purer energy. I thank the universe or God for the healing, and the pet patient, before coming fully back into consciousness. To me, it's as important as 'earthing' the physical body, mentally reminding yourself of your roots and taking a moment to acclimatize again. I always offer my client a drink of water and take a sip myself in recognition of the journey we've just been through.

Nature's Medicine Cabinet

The metaphysical aspect of healing was fascinating to me after years of working in the pharmaceutical industry, where science is king. But my inner scientist was itching to join me on my steep learning curve towards becoming an animal healer.

Ask any scientist and he or she will tell you that most experiments are based on observation, and I had already begun to take a new interest in my animals after my extraordinary experience with Wow. In particular, I was becoming fascinated by what the horses chose to *eat*.

I began to make notes while clearing their field of manure in the evenings. There's plenty of lush grass in my fields, but I'm very aware that wild horses would graze many acres, stocking up on a wider range of nutrients than are available in any paddock, even those properly rotated by responsible horse owners. I noticed how my mare Betty would paw at the ground to get at the mud and wondered if, for her, this was a milkshake version of the nutrients she was getting from the grass. Wow would nibble on quite specific types of grass. They would both choose carefully from the many plants on offer in the hedgerow at the edge of their field and, in the autumn, I watched as they reached out and almost sucked the rose hips off the thorny bushes, extending their lips to enclose them so that they wouldn't prick themselves on the thorns. Even though there was a water trough for them to drink from, I noticed that they preferred to drink from a muddy puddle when it rained.

I started experimenting a little. One hot summer's day, I was eating a banana in the yard and, when Betty leaned over to sniff it, I gave her a nibble. I was amazed when she gobbled up the whole thing. I saw that Wow was craning his head out of his stable to see what she was eating, so I went into the kitchen to get him one, too. Wow gobbled it up. I knew that this was unlikely to be a natural part of a horse's diet, but I thought that if sportspeople eat bananas because of the potassium and the electrolytes they contain, perhaps Betty and Wow were searching out some natural electrolytes to replace the salt they were losing in sweat. Interestingly, in winter this is not the case; the horses only seem to want banana when they are hot.

On another summer evening's poo-pick, I noticed that the horses were sniffing at the stinging nettles in the paddock. I have been interested in herbs since I was given a book by the original 17th-century herbalist, botanist and physician, Nicholas Culpepper, as a school prize, and it was already well thumbed. I had regularly enjoyed a cup of nettle tea, so

I turned to my trusty book to find that not only are nettles a natural diuretic and anti-inflammatory but also a blood tonic. A bunch a day is about as good for a horse as a bunch of watercress is for us. I make a lovely nettle omelette for myself these days, and the dogs lap up the leftovers.

The horses were only sniffing at the nettles that evening, as of course the sting is too sensitive for their mouths. But some weeks later I was chatting to the farmer down the road and he mentioned that, after he harrowed the fields, his cattle would make a beeline for the mown, dried nettles left behind after the silage had been harvested. He is one of the many farmers I have come across who put a great deal of store in the 'old ways' of the country, and so I decided to have a go at cutting some of my own nettles to see how the horses would take to them. After three days the sting had gone, the nettles were dry and crispy and the horses went mad for them. With ears forward they were whickering as if nettles were the horse equivalent of a gorgeous piece of Green & Black's chocolate. Again, according to Culpepper, nettles contain electrolytes which regulate and control fluids – just what my clever, overheated horses were seeking out.

I was drinking up as much information as I could now. I had already decided to work part time so that I could concentrate on my new studies, and was spending just four days a week flying around Europe, the UK and Ireland. The rest of the week was spent tending to the needs of my husband, my horses Betty and Wow, my Jack Russell Alf, my lovely boxer Bruce and… me! As I began to meditate more and to enjoy the peace of the countryside while observing my animals, I began to feel more and more out of place at those sales meetings, however. The more grounded I felt at home and the more appreciative I was of the beauty of the countryside on my own doorstep, the more disconnected I felt while away on business trips. It all felt so empty and pointless.

While I was competing at a show-jumping event at Hickstead, however, I found a reason to keep plugging away at my pharmaceutical publishing job. I was browsing through the books at one of the trade stalls, and there, among the books on horse training and dressage, was one on something called 'animal aromatics'. I had never heard of such a thing, but since I had been watching how interested my animals were in natural medicines, I picked it up to have a look. It was a tiny book by a woman called Caroline Ingraham, a pioneer in zoopharmacognosy, the science of animal self-medication, and from the first page I was hooked. I read it almost from cover to cover then and there!

Zoopharmacognosy, I learned, is the study of animals selecting aromatic plants and plant oils, algae, clay and other natural remedies for maintaining their health. This practice allows animals the opportunity to look after themselves, as they would in the wild. This was exactly what I had begun to notice with my own.

Caroline's thesis was based on the fact that animals use their sense of smell much more than we do, selecting for themselves what they need for imbalances in the body or mind as well as to stay healthy. The human olfactory bulb has shrunk in size as we have evolved, while animals still have the olfactory bulbs that they had thousands of years ago.

Since time began, animals have been self-selecting herbal remedies, and instinct still tells them what works. We have six million sensory receptors, while the average dog has between 200 and 300 million. A bloodhound has 350 million. An animal's sense of smell is its primary sense; penguins use it to find their young, dogs and cats use it to mark their territory, and sniffing is the first greeting for most animals. In the wild, sniffing the air can be the difference between life and death.

I was aware of a well-documented trial by Dr Eloy Rodriguez and Richard Wrangham, together with the famous chimpanzee expert Jane Goodall, that had studied primates' innate ability to self-select plants. I was particularly fascinated by a plant they used to control internal parasites. Primates had been observed plucking this toilet brush-shaped plant and ingesting it whole – including its sticky bristle-shaped leaves. As the plant travelled through the stomach and digestive tract, it picked up internal parasites and worms. The primates then excreted the whole plant intact, covered in worms and parasites. This was Nature's own self-wormer! I was fascinated. I just had to meet Caroline Ingraham.

It didn't take long to find her – I think her number was even on the book itself, and I rang her as soon as I got home. When she told me about the courses that she teaches in zoopharmacognosy, I was grateful that my pharmaceuticals job had provided me the money to sign up for one. I was even more thrilled to find that I would be working with animal patients on this course. At that point I had only observed my dogs and horses, but now I would be meeting all sorts of species to find out just what they would do to treat their own illnesses if they were in the wild.

I found the two-year course absolutely fascinating. I was meeting cats, dogs, horses, small furries (guinea pigs, hamsters, gerbils, etc.) and even snakes, and discovering how they respond to a wide variety of oils, plants, algae and clays.

A light bulb had gone on in me and I couldn't wait to start treating animals myself. With most complementary therapies, the therapist has to clock up a certain number of case histories, assignments and clinical hours to gain experience before setting up professionally. I took this as the perfect opportunity to offer my skills to just about anyone I could find.

I hadn't even left the course in Hay-on-Wye before I found my first patients. I had been looking around at the beautiful farmlands around me and wondering whether farm animals would self-select in the same way as some of the animals Caroline had introduced us to had done. While we were working at a small animal rescue centre in Hay, I had asked Sarah, the manager, if she knew of any farm animals that might need healing and she told me that her friend, Siobhan, ran a rescue centre in nearby Brecon where there was a Vietnamese pot-bellied pig who could do with some animal aromatic healing. I had never worked on a pig before, and jumped at the chance!

Siobhan and Lydia

I got straight on the phone to Siobhan, who told me that she was worried about the pig, whose name was Lydia. They had always enjoyed a very close relationship, but recently Lydia had begun to spend all her time in her stable, refusing even to root around outside or play with her companions. I could tell that Siobhan was very concerned, and I arranged to see her as soon as I could.

As I drove up to the farm where the rescue centre was based, I was greeted by Siobhan and a pack of waggy-tailed rescue dogs who showed me straight to Lydia's stable. I walked in with my box of oils and saw Lydia at the back of the stable, her back towards us, head down. I could feel her pain as she stood silently, not even turning to see who was coming in to see her.

I gently set my box down beside her and offered Siobhan the oils to give to her. Siobhan knew from her dealings with Caroline that only professional therapists who have trained in zoopharmacognosy over the two-year course should work with these oils, but I made sure that she offered the oils one by one, never mixing them together or adding them to food or water. It's so important to allow animals to self-select, to let them use the oils to help uncover their real health issues.

Most plant oils I use are macerated or steeped in a base oil such as sunflower or olive oil. The fresh herbs such as calendula, chickweed, nettle, mint and rose hip are macerated for a number of weeks if cold pressed, or heated gently for four hours and allowed to cool before the plant material is sieved, leaving the macerated or infused oil.

Even the base oil is produced in the traditional and natural way by gently squeezing it out of the seed at temperatures below 40°C, which ensures that the full essence and character of the oil are preserved. Once the oil has settled, it is filtered to guarantee its purity, then bottled. There is no heating or refining process, just pure healthy oil.

The plant oils have to be macerated so that they can be safely ingested. This is the traditional way that we use to store our herbs and plants, a kind of pickling process that keeps them fresh. It's important that the animal has an opportunity to choose both base oil and plant oil before I make the mixture up, and I make sure that both are the highest quality products.

This is the difference between the kind of essential oils that you can buy off the shelves and the plant oils I work with. It's dangerous to ingest an essential oil without adding a base oil – something which only trained practitioners are allowed to do.

I started with neroli. Lydia grabbed the bottle in her mouth, took several licks from the oil on Siobhan's finger, and squeaked. We watched as she sniffed it up through the limbic system, the part of the brain that processes emotion, and gave a heavy sigh of relief.

I next gave Siobhan the rose otto to offer Lydia and she sniffed it, paused, thinking very deeply as I put a drop on Siobhan's finger. Lydia licked it, but we both felt that she seemed to prefer the neroli. She licked some seaweed-and-chickweed macerated oil, which is packed with vital nutrients like minerals and trace elements and some comfrey, but turned away from both the carrot seed (which is for loss of appetite and to help liver function) and the benzoin (for deep emotional trauma).

After Lydia had clearly made her choice of the oils, I asked Siobhan if she might be grieving. The oils she had been attracted to, the neroli in particular, are for grief and the aftermath of being separated from a companion. Siobhan looked amazed and told me that several months ago Lydia had lost her beloved sister Maggie to meningitis.

Siobhan explained a little about their relationship and how Lydia had refused to bond with any of the other pigs since Maggie's death. She had also turned her back on the close friendship she had had with Siobhan.

I began to settle Lydia into a healing, with Siobhan sitting quietly beside her. I attuned myself, and Lydia soon became very relaxed and very quiet. She sank into her body, her muscles relaxed, her eyelids heavy, and soon she was snoring peacefully. When I had finished the healing, she was quite a different pig. She walked over to Siobhan, chortling quietly, her tail spinning like a helicopter. It was clear that they had a very special bond and Siobhan was in tears as she hugged her old friend. I'm always astonished at how quickly self-selection of healing oils seems to have an effect. It is as if the limbic system deals with all the pain immediately. The oils clearly touch a nerve, but instead of triggering a negative reaction, emotions are released. The animal seems to feel listened to, and often that's enough. If only it were that easy for the rest of us!

As humans we can let our emotions out by crying, and even though many of us feel embarrassed about showing our emotions and hold that stress in the body, we can let it go with a good cry. Animals have tear ducts, too, but they can't express their grief in quite the same way. Just like us, they too can bottle up frustration and pain, and this sometimes reveals itself in behavioural problems such as aggression or deeply upset or subdued behaviour.

Lydia and Biddy

Siobhan was thrilled with Lydia's recovery and asked me if I would go and see Biddy, a 13-year-old pot-bellied pig who had recently recovered from meningitis. I was thrilled at the opportunity to meet another animal and I wondered how many others Siobhan would introduce me to while I was at her rescue centre.

Biddy lived alone in a sty at the other end of the farm. She was an entirely different character to Lydia; in fact she reminded me of Hattie Jakes, the bossy matron in the *Carry On* films. She was much more irritable than Lydia and lived separately from her to avoid fights breaking out between them. She had already trashed Lydia's home. I handed Siobhan some of the neroli and rose otto which Lydia had gobbled up, but Biddy showed little interest. She also turned down the yarrow, an anti-inflammatory and analgesic which I thought she might need at 13 years old with the inevitable stiffening of joints. She also turned up her snout at the garlic, a blood tonic and immune stimulant; I had wondered if she could be harbouring a virus which might be making her irritable and run down. The highly nutritious chickweed and melissa, so often the favourite among female animals, were also not of any interest to her. But as soon as Biddy was offered vanilla pod steeped in sunflower oil, she grabbed the bottle and drank the equivalent of two small mugs! Fresh vanilla pod is marvellous at balancing the female hormones; it seemed that Biddy was just a middle-aged lady suffering from a bit of menopausal crankiness!

Next I handed some nutmeg (which I had brought over from Grenada) to Siobhan to offer to Biddy. One of nutmeg's properties is to mimic the female hormone oestrogen and it can balance unpredictable scattered energies. Biddy gobbled it up, confirming my initial thoughts. By the next day Lydia and Biddy were outside together, getting on happily. Siobhan still kept them in separate sties, with a small wall dividing them, but they were able to sniff each other, snout to snout.

Jake the Rat

Siobhan took me into the house for a cup of tea and, as we sat in her kitchen, I noticed a beautiful pet rat sitting in his cage in the corner of the room. Rats make excellent pets and are extremely intelligent, often recognizing their own name after only a couple of days. I was immediately drawn to Jake's expressive eyes. I felt sick as Siobhan told me how she had rescued him after a tip-off that he was being badly abused by his owner, and as she showed me the cigarette-burn scars which he had been the victim of, I found it hard to fight back the tears. I hadn't met many rescue animals by this stage in my animal healing career. Sadly, I'm more used to them these days.

Jake seemed to be such a sweet, intelligent animal and I couldn't bear to think of what he had suffered. I let him sniff some rose otto to help him release some of the physical and psychological trauma. I always offer this one first; the healing process for animals will always start by a release of the emotions, just as it does for us. I was just beginning my journey into zoopharmacognosy at the time, but I still have never seen an animal become so obsessed with an essential oil. Jake grabbed the bottle in his mouth, his little paws clutching it as if he just couldn't get enough. I managed to prise it out of his grasp and put a few drops onto a dish, which he licked clean. He then perched on his hind legs, clearly asking for more. He must have been holding so much pain in his little body, and this was his way of letting some of it go. I had no idea how much rose otto he would take.

I had spotted a rose bush in full bloom outside and I asked Siobhan if I could go and get some to put in a vase next to Jake. She readily agreed, and as we placed the flowers on a little table right next to Jake's cage, he stood up on his back legs and poked his nose into the flower heads, drinking in the smell. Finally sitting back, he curled his little body up and looked lost in thought, clearly processing some very deep memories. As rats have poor eyesight, they rely heavily on their sense of smell and the petals seemed to give him comfort, like a favourite blanket can be to a small child. I made up a remedy of rose otto in spring water and gave Siobhan instructions for how to administer it to Jake.

A couple of months later Siobhan phoned to give me an update on her animals. Lydia was still very content and occasionally wanting a sniff of neroli while Biddy, although far less moody, was occasionally taking the vanilla pod. But Jake was still suffering. He had done so well in his rehabilitation in the smaller cage that Siobhan had decided he could go into a bigger space. A rat cage should have enough space and sufficient height for climbing and plenty of toys to play with, and Siobhan had given Jake a beautiful new one with lovely cardboard bedding. She had made sure that none of it was chemically treated to avoid any respiratory problems, but despite her care and attention, Jake had curled into a ball and refused to come out of his little house. It was almost as if he were suffering from agoraphobia.

When I was next completing another module at Hay-on-Wye, I went back to see Jake and asked Siobhan to offer him the oils again. This time he self-selected violet leaf, which has many remedial properties including those for new surroundings and nervousness, but he wasn't interested in the rose at all. He seemed to need more than the oils and I decided to do a full healing on him.

I sat down in one of Siobhan's comfy armchairs and placed Jake on my lap. He was curious at first to explore, but soon settled down as I focused on grounding the energies and sending him wave after wave of pure unconditional love. He stretched out on my lap and gently closed his eyes. My hands slightly apart and spanning most of his body, I could feel him absorbing the energy.

After the healing, Jake woke up and immediately started to groom himself, feeling totally happy with where he was. I put him back in his cage and he seemed to have a new confidence as he explored it. I gave thanks to God and to Jake himself, and felt that my work was done. Siobhan phoned me later to tell me that Jake was readily accepting cuddles from the family, and I appreciated more than ever the power of spiritual healing and how this would always form the backbone of all of my animal healing work.

The Business of Plants

After seeing the effect of healing and plant oils on Jake the rat and the pot-bellied pigs, I knew that Nature had a great deal more to teach me and I couldn't wait to plant my own garden and open a clinic where I could treat animals with home-grown plant material. Years later, my herb garden is one of the first things that many of my clients notice as they pull into my drive. People tell me that the lovely hedgerows lining the lane to my clinic are enough to transport them away from the white coats and scanning machines of their vet surgeries, as they realize that this is a place where medicine grows in the garden. The smell of mint, calendula, comfrey, lavender, bay, catnip, yarrow and lemon balm, mixed with the natural smells of the countryside, greets them as they walk past the stable yard.

I have always been drawn to indigenous plant materials, especially those growing in the UK which I had learnt about from my Culpepper book at school. Herbs and plants were more than just medicine to me; from my early teens I was interested in cooking with culinary herbs, and my mother and I loved to experiment with rosemary and bay leaf stuffed in a chicken, or with fresh thyme scattered over the skin.

Mealtimes were the only time I would see my father, who worked hard all day, so cooking for the family and sitting down to eat with them was very special and I would use herbs in just about everything I put down in front of them. I loved the smell of basil with tomato or even a cup of mint tea from the garden. I was fascinated by textures, too; while all my school friends were chewing spearmint gum, I was chewing raw mint leaves! My breath smelled great and my concentration levels soared, especially during end-of-year exams.

By my mid-twenties I had already gathered a vast knowledge about plants while working in medical publishing, which was particularly helpful when I began training in zoopharmacognosy and self-selection. I was still whizzing off to conferences on prescriptive drugs and their uses for part of the week, and healing sick animals during the other half, building a deep understanding of how science borrows from Nature. I realized that most drugs are synthetically cloned from Nature's own medicine cabinet. Digitalis, for example, the drug often used for heart conditions, is derived from the foxglove, and aspirin is derived from salicylates, which come from the willow species, and has been known since ancient times for its medicinal properties. Horses will often tuck into willow leaf to medicate themselves if it is available in the field or hedgerows.

I had followed the growth in interest in herbal remedies over the years, watching the balance shift between what science is capable of and what the natural world can offer, so I was thrilled to be part of the pharmaceutical industry at a time when the use of natural plant medicines was becoming a growing trend.

One of my biggest clients was based in Vienna and worked with mainstream companies like Eli Lilly, a giant amongst the pharmaceutical industry. Prozac, now a very well-known antidepressant, was one of its global best sellers and is a synthetic version of the hormone serotonin which we manufacture naturally in the brain. Eli Lilly recognized that the natural plant St John's wort was becoming a very serious competitor, as it appeared to work in the same way as many of the most successful antidepressants, by inhibiting the re-uptake of serotonin in the brain. The remedial properties of St John's wort are well documented now and it can be bought in supermarkets these days, but at that time it was a revelation that it could help with depression. This was the 21st-century pharmaceutical industry meeting 17th-century Culpepper, and I loved it.

Now the industry is changing yet again. As strains of bacteria become more aggressive and mutate, scientists are finding it increasingly difficult to keep up with the demand for new drugs to combat infectious diseases, and are finding many of the answers by observing animals self-selecting plants in the wild. This is a brand-new apothecary of plant medicines, and what I love is that after so many years of animal experiments, it means that the mentors in science are now the animals themselves.

I was so excited by this. I could sniff the winds of change and I knew that it would take my career in a totally new direction. As the demand for complementary healthcare was growing for humans, so it was for animals. More and more pet owners were recognizing that although the vet is always the first port of call, there had to be more to getting well than pills alone. If complementary therapies worked for humans, would it be such a leap of faith to try them on pets?

This had become my mission. I really felt that I had experienced some kind of epiphany while healing Wow, and studying zoopharmacognosy had fulfilled a childhood dream. I had an inner knowing, a gut feeling that this was my future.

I busily continued, travelling all over the country and adding letters to my name for the next six years, using my part-time publishing job to fund professional courses. Everything I had achieved so far had been through hard work and focus. I was methodical, grounded and, perhaps because of my parents' combination of unconditional love and a rigorous work ethic, I totally believed in myself. Even though I was still only in my early thirties, I had a strong sense of my life falling into place. That ambition I had had at the *Daily Mail*, that intense sense of purpose I had had when first healing my broken horse fuelled a feeling of destiny, of finding something that was truly me. Now I was also graced with a passion for creating a clinic at my home with its own apothecary of herbs harvested from my own garden. It was fantastically fulfilling.

A Clinic Is Born

I had already started to build up a small practice healing friends' animals in my upstairs room, and word had begun to spread. When a local newspaper ran an article on my unusual combination of healing and plant oils, it elicited hundred of calls which translated into enough new patients for me to give up my publishing job and throw myself completely into the work I was born to do.

My plan was taking form. I would set up the first full-time animal healing clinic specializing in hands-on healing, distant healing and plant self-selection as well as advice about diet and environment. Uniquely, I would be able to offer pet owners healing, counselling and behaviour training as well, something that I couldn't believe no one else in the whole country was offering. It seemed to me that the relationship between owner and pet was crucial in the treatment of most of the issues I had already seen, and as my studies had equipped me with these skills as part of the holistic therapy, I was excited at what lay ahead. As news travelled, the phone was already ringing off the hook.

I already knew that I couldn't do this on my own for long. I remember feeling so inspired and motivated when I finished my healing courses that I told my teacher that I wanted to go and heal the world. He put his hand on my shoulder and gently reminded me to make sure that I was using my energy properly. He advised me not to spread myself too thinly if I didn't want to burn out. I remember thinking then that if I could teach others to do the same work with healing, maybe we could heal the world between us. So I set about designing a diploma course in animal healing, which now attracts a steadily growing number of students. For more information, see www.healinganimals.org

All the healers listed here have successfully graduated from the one-year Animal Healing Diploma with Elizabeth Whiter and for the equine healers an additional six-month course was completed. These unique courses involved intensive study, training and practical experience. All these graduates have demonstrated dedication, compassion and a loving ability to offer healing to animals and their carers. The high standards achieved by these graduates are a result of their hard work, the professional teaching staff and the vigorous assessment and written examinations required by the external examiner.
DIANE RAINBOW-TOWERS, MPHIL, BA (HONS), DIPCG, DIPHE.

Hazel and Shauny

One of my first students was a woman who helped me take my plan to the next stage.

I couldn't wait to plant my own herb garden and start stocking my own apothecary, but I needed help and, fittingly, it was a cat who brought it to my door. These days, Hazel is an 'intuitive gardener' and has an allotment where she seeds some of my plants, especially the calendula, and organizes plant sales to raise money for animals in need and my own Healing Animals Organisation. She is a graduate of my diploma course in animal healing and already has her own client base, yet when I met her she was in a stressful job in financial services and was clearly not happy. She reminded me of myself when I was in medical publishing and feeling so out of sorts with the commercial world. She seemed to know that there was more to life, something more fulfilling to do. She wanted to be of service.

Her cat Shauny had an overactive thyroid gland and Hazel, on hearing about my work, had brought him to see me. Shauny was a beautiful fawn tabby with huge yellow eyes. Hazel called him her 'paper tiger' because he seemed big and butch to those he was comfortable with, but with strangers he was very shy.

Shauny and his sister Shelley had been rescued as kittens from a sanctuary back in 1991 and had a wonderful life and a great relationship with Hazel. Shauny was Hazel's constant companion, and she believed that his love and loyalty had been a significant factor in her successful recovery from pneumonia.

When they first came to see me, Shauny was suffering from vomiting and weight loss, despite an increased appetite, and irritability. He had been diagnosed with hyperthyroidism a year before, and Hazel had given him the prescribed medication for several weeks until the side effects became unacceptable and she had made the difficult decision to cancel the medicine. With the help of flower remedies and homeopathy he had stabilized, but his enormous appetite meant that he needed food every few hours – and lots of it.

Despite Shauny's anxiety with strangers, when he arrived in the clinic he came straight out of the basket and had a good look around the room and a good sniff. Hazel was amazed at how he took to me as if he had known me all his life. He purred and rubbed himself up against me, loving the healing and relaxing deeply. Hazel too found the experience a wonderful relief after a year of worry.

By his second session, Shauny was enjoying the healing so much that I cut and dried some catnip for him and encouraged him to roll in it in a large tray. Catnip is a feline euphoric, an antispasmodic sedative which helps calm nerves and promote restful sleep. It is the aroma of the nepetalactone that cats become intoxicated with, and I use this herb to help stressed rescue cats acclimatize to their new surroundings at sanctuaries both here and abroad.

Shauny looked like a sphinx as he sat in the tray, so majestic and proud. Hazel was mesmerized by this newly confident stance as he purred loudly and looked me straight in the eye, tapping his tail on the stone floor. She had never seen him like this before.

He began to roll in his tray and seemed to be loving his catnip spa, so I suggested that Hazel lie on the couch and accept a healing. She was so tired, and gladly accepted the offer. Shauny, refreshed from his aromatherapy, curled up on the tiled floor under the desk, keeping a watchful eye on both of us and providing his own meditative sound by purring throughout our healing session.

It is the most satisfying feeling when I witness pet and owner blissed out and completely at one. It really brings home to me the incredible bond we share with our beloved friends from the animal kingdom, and I am so grateful to have such wonderful people and animals finding their way to me.

As we chatted later over a cup of tea, Hazel wanted to know everything about healing. She seemed to be looking at ways in which she could change her life. She had recently been made redundant, and this had left her scared of the unknown. I encouraged her to see it as the breakthrough she needed, how when things appear to go wrong they are often an opportunity to create positive thoughts and manifest what we actually do want in our lives.

She told me about her passion for plants, flowers and vegetables, and an idea began to emerge. Her vision of creating a harmonious relationship between people, animals and plants living together as organically as possible and honouring the natural cycles and laws of life was one I shared. I was so attracted to her enthusiasm that I asked her to help me design my herb garden.

The Herb Garden

It has become one of my greatest pleasures in life. I love to spend hours planting, weeding and harvesting, with the dogs pottering about beside me, and as I do I often think fondly of Shauny, who died aged 15, a year after he first came to see me. His sister Shelley was diagnosed with the same condition that same year, but Hazel's experience of healing and self-medication meant that this time she was more confident about the prognosis. She managed to administer the prescribed medication, wrapped in a small piece of cheese spread, despite the side effect of vomiting, and balanced the allopathic treatment with healings as well as with a new home-cooked diet. Shelley's stomach problems have since reduced, and she is still alive at 17 and leading a happy (and very spoiled) life.

My herb garden is a wonderful little eco-system right under my nose, and it reminds me every day of the delicate balance of life on earth. I deliberately planted comfrey, feverfew, garlic, chives, lavender, mint and yarrow to attract the right insects such as ladybirds and spiders, as well as the many little birds which eat the aphids and midges.

The herb garden is near the stables, where a family of swallows nests. Of course the stables are the perfect habitat for insects, which in turn make a feast for the swallows. We have a flourishing bird population in the garden, including owls, which are an essential part of the eco-system here as they eat the pest insects. I don't use any form of insecticide, but I do find that crushed eggshells around certain plants are a great deterrent to slugs.

My lovely friend Reg Lanaway is a passionate ornithologist and has been helping me to ring swallows for four years. Although he is in his early seventies, he is still lecturing at Plumpton Agricultural College and observes for The Royal Society for the Protection of Birds to track birds' longevity and migration routes. This year alone we have ringed over 50 baby swallows and have been amazed to find that their families come back to us from South Africa each year, remaking their little nests out of hay, mud and shavings from the horses' stable and yard. They perch in the eaves in the stables; when I give healing to Wow I have a sea of little faces watching me.

I harvest my own herbs anywhere between late May and August. I need five days of dry, sunny weather, and as the British summer is so unpredictable I never know for sure what I'm going to be able to harvest. Too much rain can so easily destroy the whole crop. I always examine the herbs to feel how dry they are, and over the years I have had to abandon many harvested herbs like mint and comfrey because damp conditions can allow mildew to develop.

I pick only from noon onwards as this is the best time to release the precious oils in the plants, and as long as the weather is good it's great to be able to put my shorts on and spend a couple of hours sitting with my basket and my scissors after a morning in the clinic. Surrounded by the incredible colours of the calendula and lavender, the magic of Nature never fails to inspire me.

Nothing is wasted in the garden; even the mildewed herbs are put on the compost heap. I cut nettles and dry them until the sting is gone and then use them as a mild anti-inflammatory and diuretic. I'll be honest, though; harvesting my own herbs is a labour of love and I really don't envy farmers their work. For the scale of my needs, it would take so much more time than I have. But it's such a wonderful feeling to have grown them myself and to sit among them that I never tire of it. It never ceases to amaze me when my seemingly barren herb garden suddenly bursts into life. Gardening is such a lovely meditative thing to do, and it thrills me that I can use it as part of my healing.

I use the manure from my own horses, which are fed an organic alfalfa horse feed that is high in proteins, enzymes and amino acids and contains vitamins A, B_1, B_2, C and K as well as potassium, magnesium, copper, cobalt and iron, minerals and vitamins that horses would naturally get from their grasses in the wild. It also means that the herbs themselves are organic.

My window sills are packed with over 250 aloe vera plants throughout the summer. The leaves are so useful that I bought a separate freezer to freeze them for the winter months. I often go to rescue centres after the best of the aloe season, so I defrost them and make them into a topical base to take with me. I've got a whole medicine cabinet on my garden sills at the moment, infusing in the natural sunshine. I'll leave St John's wort, borage, calendula and chickweed for a clear five days of sunshine, bringing them in if it rains, until the sun shines again.

When I'm not harvesting them from my own garden, I buy as much as I can from an organic supplier. I need to be absolutely sure of the quality of products I buy in for my animal patients; if I can't use my own herbs I try to get as much organic material as I can. Sometimes, however, this isn't possible – the seaweed I buy, for instance, is hand-harvested from the French Atlantic, and since nothing from the sea can be certified organic, I can't claim that my apothecary is 100 per cent organic.

My apothecary is filled with my herbs and plant material along with blenders and measuring jugs, weighing scales, large metal saucepans, sieves and funnels for the macerated plant oils. The shelves are covered in tightly lidded glass containers packed with herbs, clays, spirulina, flower heads, hips and plant material. It's important to preserve them in a dry environment so that they don't deteriorate, and most will last in these jars for up to a year.

I love to potter about in the apothecary and I take my clients in there to offer them a home-grown mint. Many of my clients regularly use herbal teas and understand the remedial properties of the most common herbs such as St John's wort and chamomile. They may not have thought of using them on their animals before, but they don't need to be persuaded once the connection is made. I make sure, too, that they realize that offering macerated oils to an animal is *not* a substitute for a vet's prescription.

As we chat I'll pass on tips about how to use herbs at home to help with their pet's condition and which will complement the vet's prescription. I've always loved playing around with different recipes since I first devoured my Culpepper book at school, and I have discovered all sorts of wonderful herbal recipes. I use calendula flowers with a small pinch of sea salt in boiling water for a particularly good eyewash which I allow to cool and then use to bathe around the eyes. Green clay infused with peppermint, or aloe and peppermint together, is fabulous for soothing any itching after a day in the herb garden. Garlic is a wonderful antimicrobial that helps to kill parasites, and seaweed clay is a great toothpaste for animals, particularly cats with gingivitis. Manuka honey is fabulous for shock and trauma as well as a great natural antibiotic, and cranberry is a wonderful treatment for urinary tract infections. Neem oil helps to repel fleas and to heal skin irritations. For many centuries Indians have used the seeds, bark and leaves of this impressive insect repellent on themselves and their animals and as <u>an antiviral, antiseptic, antifungal</u> <u>remedy.</u>

All the herbs I grow can be used in various forms. I infuse them for myself as teas, or give them to the animals just as they are or as macerated oils, simmered gently in olive oil for over four hours. My kitchen smells gorgeous when I've got a brew of calendula heads on the hob and some rose leaf syrup just out of the pan. After they come off the heat, I'll blend the sludge and sieve the herbs, which I then use for a whole host of things. I make a fabulous vinaigrette from the calendula heads with a dash of balsamic vinegar and more olive oil, and I make the best night cream from the calendula heads heated in a bain-marie with fresh local beeswax. It makes a bit of an orange mess of my pillowcases, but I love what it does for my skin.

Nature's Rewards

I always tell clients who have seen what native herbs can offer their animals how important it is to give something back. Understanding the benefits of plant life raises their consciousness about the countryside and what we can do to avoid its decline.

The downside of the explosion of interest in herbs has meant that many plants are becoming over-exploited, and some are even near extinction. Like so many of our other natural resources, many plants are being plundered in our passion for consumption and we are forgetting to give them back to Mother Earth. There are now no fewer than 345 wild plants in Britain struggling for survival, according to the Vascular Plant Red Data List for Britain, published in May 2007. The list was compiled by the JNCC (Joint Nature Conservation Committee), the conservation charity Plantlife, the Botanical Society for the British Isles, the Biological Records Centre, the Countryside Council for Wales, English Nature, Royal Botanic Garden Edinburgh, Scottish Natural Heritage and the Natural History Museum.

Many of these plants are being polluted by the soil itself after years of agricultural fertilizers and intensive farming methods as well as the impact of car exhaust fumes, factory waste and air pollution – all of which are man-made. Plants are being overfed a junk-food diet of fertilizers and sewage, and those that do survive have little nutritional or medicinal value. Aggressive weeds such as giant hogweed are now growing up to six feet high and poisoning the soil for some of the smaller plants with valuable medicinal properties.

Farmers and smallholders used to be the caretakers of the natural world, but many are now using former grasslands, traditionally a home for wild plants, for animals such as deer or sheep to over-graze. Some modern farming methods have led to the destruction of hedgerows, causing the loss of valuable herbs such as hawthorn, rose, dogwood, crab apple and holly, and of non-climbers found in hedgerows such as primrose, red campion and stitchwort.

My friends and colleagues from the farming community are all committed guardians of the countryside and are right behind the new Environmental Stewardship scheme introduced by the government in March 2007, which encourages farmers to tend the land in ways that are friendly to wildlife. They are now being offered cash incentives to revive the age-old tradition of looking after hedgerows, which provide a habitat for birds and small animals, and creating areas of wildflowers for bees and other beneficial insects. They are being asked to protect ponds from pesticides and fertilizers to try and halt the decline in frog and newt numbers and encourage wild birds to nest here.

I find it very sad that so much of the natural way of the countryside has been interfered with and that supermarkets in particular have transformed the relationship between farmer and consumer. Being forced to produce milk and meat for the cheapest prices has meant that so many of our farmers have been driven out of the business, and farms themselves are being sold off as residential and commercial housing. Many farmers have to diversify and convert their barns into business units. At least the growth in farm shops and educational trips has been one diversification that has benefited the wider community.

Others have managed to salvage something from the crisis. My farmer friend Michael Best, who supplies my hay, couldn't afford to carry on with his dairy business and, much as he loved his cows, he had to give up the herd after generations of dairy farming in his family. But Michael was at least able to give in to his other great love and create natural habitats for wildlife out of his pasture land. Now it is woodland and a haven of beauty. Native trees such as oak, beech, hawthorn and birch and wild grasses now provide a grassland track around the edge of the woodland, making it into a paradise for horse riders. I often ride here at dawn and lose myself in the tranquillity of the place. It's a wonderful start to the day to be able to see barn owls, buzzards, kestrels, rabbits and, if I'm lucky, a family of deer. I ride home intoxicated by the delicious smells of honeysuckle and dog rose from the hedgerows, inspired and ready for my day in the clinic.

Instinct and Intuition

One of the most gratifying things about what I do is witnessing the moment when the intellect of the mind surrenders to the wisdom of the heart, the moment when reason is put aside and something quite magical happens.

When an owner watches his pet selecting a remedy for her cancer, a macerated oil for her fear of being alone, or rolling over to allow her aching hip to be healed by my hands, the owner is usually humbled by this instinct, and the relationship between them is transformed.

In terms of real knowledge we've got nothing on most of the dogs, cats, rats, guinea pigs and horses I see, yet we're supposed to be top of the food chain. We only need to watch the way our animals live to observe how their intuition, their ability to tune in to energies, their instincts are all finely honed. Our animals remind us to think less and chill out more. They know what's what. They know whom to follow, how to lead, even what to eat to make themselves healthy.

Spending as much time as I do with those who live in harmony with their environment, whose carbon footprint contributes so little to climate change and whose belief system melts hearts rather than creates wars, I'm often left scratching my head about our modern world.

One of the problems with modern education is that it teaches us that science is king. I'm fascinated by science, but it is based on solutions and can't prove most of the things that I see every day. To modern science, anecdotal evidence is inadmissible, so witnessing results counts for nothing according to its rigorous methodology.

Happily, as far as my clients are concerned we see all the results we need.

Most vets I come across are very respectful of the work that I do and see it as complementing theirs. I love the fact that I can combine knowledge of the endocrine system with intuition around the energy centres, taking the best of both worlds in my work. The physiology and anatomy module is one of the cornerstones of my animal healing course, yet the body is only half the story when we're dealing with a living being.

Vets work with animals because they have a deep understanding of what they are, and apply their scientific minds to animals' wellbeing. But I find that veterinary training and dedication create a certain mindset which does not allow them to expand their thinking. As with all modern medicine, time is at a premium and vets, like doctors, don't have enough of it to look under the surface or to tune intuitively in to the source of the problem. One thing that scientists/doctors and vets agree on is that the most effective remedy is the *time* that complementary therapists can spend on their patients.

Things are changing, though: veterinary schools in Europe and the US are beginning to invite specialist complementary therapists to lecture their students, and the final year at some veterinary schools offers students an opportunity to explore complementary healthcare such as acupuncture and herbalism.

I have deep respect for the enormous advances in medicine, but being around animals can teach us a great deal. Animals are deeply empowering for us, especially when they mirror our emotions. They can be great healers, and the moment when their owners wake up to the real relationship their pets can offer is a profound one indeed.

I believe that it is part of our role as top of the food chain to be good leaders and to understand the needs of everybody else on Earth if we're to keep ourselves and our planet healthy. It is about moving out of the master/servant relationship into a deeper understanding of the primal bond between humans and animals. Understanding and respecting the needs of the animal kingdom is about understanding and respecting yourself, your environment and the vital role you play in others' lives.

I don't see animals as anything less than our equals. The idea that a cat is less important than a human because of the size of its brain is mad to me; watch him stalk his prey as effortlessly as a lion, without any real need to do so, and tell me who is master of his universe. Because humanity has figured out how to build motorways and travel to the moon, are we superior? Look at the way we raise chickens in battery farms, transport pigs in appalling conditions across Europe and think we're getting value for money when we buy cheap meat at the supermarket. Does that make us top of the food chain or uncivilized animal abusers?

Our survival skills, once so dependent on our instincts, are sharpened by logic and strategy these days, and the good old gut seems an uncomfortable place to look for answers. We've become too evolved for our own good. We use new head-based skills to find our answers, and place little regard on what, deep down, we know to be true.

Brain Training

We were given two sides to our brains: the right, more intuitive brain and the left, more logical brain. So why shouldn't we use them both? I host meditation and healing evenings once a month that offer training for the right brain, a natural way of increasing our intuition. For me, meditation is the greatest workout I can do. It opens up my mind and gives me the feeling that God is in me. Everyone is searching for something and I find that, as I get older, I've never felt so comfortable in my own skin. The connection with something higher is like a validation from the universe that love is all it's about. It's about being content. Even if there are testing things going on in my life, I find that I can work through them, seeing the challenges as gifts.

My healing meditation evenings attract an enormous variety of people of all ages and backgrounds, but my favourites are when we have a mix of vets, doctors and spiritual healers, farmers and my animal healing students and graduates.

I love the way that they talk about spleen function and diet in the same breath as energy blocks in the endocrine system, energy centres and animal communication when they're healing that evening's animal guests. It's a huge task for people to surrender their left brain, to stop asking 'Why?', but they come month after month because they find that when you operate from your heart, there are no more questions.

Many of them are former or current clients of mine who knew very little about healing or meditation before they came to me but have seen the effects in their own lives and want more. After they have tapped back into their real needs through their animals, they often feel so empowered that they make fundamental changes to their lifestyles. Some join my course and become healers themselves.

We meet once a month. It's a good place for like-minded souls to network among their peer groups, for holistic therapists and friends to share their experiences. After a brief introduction around the circle, I take everyone through a guided meditation. To the soundtrack of one of the healing CDs I produce with my sister, I guide them through the attunement, grounding them deeply. This is a wonderful opportunity to still the mind before we focus on the animals brought to the group for healing. It is so important that everyone lets go of any anxieties so we that we can create a group consciousness. Sometimes we focus our healing on the animals who can't get to the group, through distant healing. It's wonderful to have such a rich mix of people and experience there, and to realize that love is all you need to heal.

Once our focus is back in the room and we have shared our meditative journeys, we get to work on the animals. I love meditation and the inner peace that it restores, but it's quite another thing to be able to focus that beautiful energy and use it to heal an animal in distress.

On one typical evening, the group was gathered around several pets: Boo, a young dog whose high temperature and listless behaviour had foxed all the vets, Poppy the springer rescued from a puppy farm whose pups were taken too early and who was now feeding two rescue terrier pups, Frankie and Benny the rat brothers, one of whom was suffering from cancer, and Jinx the beautiful Siamese cat, who suffers from an overactive thyroid.

Some members of the group were spiritual healers and were picking up on the animals' emotions, while others were students of mine happy to practise what they have learned on the course. Others were simply drinking up the lovely serenity that this focused meditation brings to the middle of the Sussex countryside on a Tuesday evening.

As the animals began to relax, Poppy rolled onto her back to allow full access to her heart centre where she had experienced so much grief, while Boo snoozed happily as Alison, a GP and one of my graduate healers, conducted a beautiful healing on her. Frankie and Benny both soaked up the attention, releasing the anxieties that sibling pets always feel when one is ill. Jinx had become fixated on John, a lovely man in his late fifties who had only recently discovered meditation and who was now clearly blissed out. Animals are like sponges and soak up our energy, and Jinx was bathing in John's glow, head-butting him gently and winding her tail around him. The rest of the group joked that the two of them should 'get a room'!

The group feel that we are accomplishing something very special on these evenings, rather than just focusing on our individual development. We feel that the more we put into something, the more we learn. As a group, we know we can raise a positive vibration, and we feel connected to each other as we do. There is no place for egos or judgements in meditation, and it's a wonderful feeling to find such a strong sense of peace and love, to know that we all share an intention to help the animals – and their companions – heal themselves.

The Doors of Perception

In my opinion, most of us think too much. Meditation is a wonderful opportunity to give our overactive brains some time off, while opening the subconscious and expanding our natural intuition. I believe that meditation develops the connection with our spirituality and opens up the doors of perception. It allows us to make better decisions for ourselves and the people and animals we love. It puts both sides of the brain into balance and helps us to live our lives more fully and with more awareness.

Animals are in tune with the rhythms of the day. They know when it's time to get up, time to eat, time for a walk. They even know what time we're coming home. Their focus is completely on their 'pack', while ours tends to be more self-centred. But with a little meditation practice we can train our intuition to expand and become more in tune with other people as well as with our animals.

Most people will have experienced the moment when they are thinking of a friend, the phone rings and it's the friend on the line, but I was amazed when I found an unlikely connection with my Jack Russell while I was on the other side of the Atlantic.

Brian and I were on honeymoon in Lake Tahoe in northern California while my sister, Susie, was at home minding the dogs. Brian was observing wildlife through his binoculars, taking in the majesty of the birds of prey and the mountains around us, while I was sitting in meditation, taking in the energy and peace of this beautiful part of the world. Suddenly I felt a trickle coming from my nose. I opened my eyes and dabbed at my nostril and found I had a nosebleed. As Brian helped me clear up with what little we had with us, we wondered what might have brought it on. Brian suggested that it might have something to do with the altitude. Brian is very grounded and practical, as am I. He's my rock and I love him for it, but I knew somehow that it wasn't anything to do with altitude.

When we got home, I told Susie my tales from Tahoe and mentioned that I had had a nosebleed while meditating by the lake. She laughed and said that it was probably in sympathy with Alf, my Jack Russell. She told me how he had come into the house with blood pouring out of his nose and she had immediately scooped him up and taken him to the vet. It turned out to be nothing more serious than a cut, and when she found the same blood on a stone covering a mouse nest near the house, she deduced that he must have nicked his nose while trying to get at the mice. It's an annual fixation of his – the mice come in from the harvest and Alfie paws and licks at it for weeks – so I knew immediately what she meant. She hadn't intended telling me anything about it as it was so inconsequential. Fascinated now, I asked her when this had happened. Alf's bleeding had been at exactly the same time as mine, despite the thousands of miles between us.

In itself, the nosebleed was meaningless. The connection was not obvious enough for me to ring home and check if anything was wrong, and Alf's cut wasn't serious enough for me to need to. But it served as a reminder for me that I am deeply connected to my animals.

It also made me realize that giving myself the space to meditate can open up my consciousness so much. My intention with my work is to be of service to humans and animals, and I love what I am doing. It is my true vocation, but I'm always busy focusing on everyone else and I rarely have time off. America and its awe-inspiring landscape is a place where we love to spend our occasional holidays. For me it is where Heaven meets Earth, where Nature overwhelms me with its power and beauty. Nature demands that those who play with it are properly grounded, and when I meditate out in the desert or canoe in the Hoover Dam amid the full wonder of the Grand Canyon, I have to take care to root myself properly so that Nature doesn't literally overwhelm me. My canoe trip down the Colorado River was a moment when I knew what surrender really meant, being at one with the magnificence of those red rocks, the deep blue of the sky and the white waters of the river, so tiny and so vulnerable in the enormity of this beautiful place. As we bobbed downstream, our guide was astonished to see a bald eagle following us, something he said he hadn't seen for seven years. It was confirmation for me that there is something deeply spiritual about Nature, while bringing us back to the very essence of what being grounded really means.

PART TWO
Tales from the Clinic

Until one has loved an animal, a part of one's soul remains unawakened.
ANATOLE FRANCE

Arrival

My consulting room looks out over the beautiful Sussex countryside. The herb garden outside wafts the most magical scent through the windows, and the sweet smell of macerating calendula from the kitchen is enough to have most animals salivating before they even get through the door.

For most animals, their sense of smell is their primary indicator of safety or danger, and as they sniff the country air in the stable yard most of my animal patients, especially those who have been before, can't wait to get into the house, and very often lead their owners in through the garden gate.

Before we start the session I always let dogs run around my own garden before taking them into the kitchen. I much prefer my lawn to be a natural habitat rather than a manicured showpiece, although we do keep the grass short so that we can enjoy the songbirds, insects and wildflowers, comfrey and feverfew plants. There are masses of rambling rose bushes heavy with flowers waiting to be picked, and it's lovely to see pets and owners relax as they drink in the atmosphere of the place.

I put my own dogs in the lounge with their toys, water and beds about five minutes before the client arrives. They love to see old friends, but it could be a bit unsettling for a new animal to meet my enthusiastic gang at the door. After an initial one-on-one consultation, and if I am satisfied that the animal can meet my dogs, I let them get together.

My two young Norfolk terriers, Morris and Lily, have become more than companions, friends and part of my family. They play a very important role in helping to rehabilitate other dogs with behaviour problems such as lack of socialization skills and pack issues. Many rescue dogs who come to me have real problems with other dogs, especially in a park or open spaces. Some have been taken away from their siblings far too early, denying them the crucial socialization stage in their development. Puppies must be with other dogs before they are 16 weeks old if they are to avoid becoming aggressive or frightened of their peers, which can make life very difficult for their owners when they want to take them out. It's not the dog's fault if he or she behaves unpredictably in public; there is no such thing as a bad animal in my book, just owners who need help with training.

A lot of my work is based on observation, and the way in which my animal patient arrives is incredibly important. I watch the way he moves and check to see if there is any lameness or something in his demeanour that could be significant. It's important to notice if a cat is sitting huddled at the back of her carrier, or if she is eager to see her new surroundings. I only allow cats out of their carriers once they are in my consultation room, but it's very telling for me to see the lead an owner will take, so I sometimes leave the owner with the cat for a while to settle in to the new surroundings if the cat is particularly nervous.

I also watch the interaction between owner and animal. Some are already apologizing for their animals, others are pulling an enthusiastic animal back on the lead, overcompensating for their animal or calming him when it's not necessary. It's lovely to see owners who talk to their animals as much as they talk to me, recognizing the equal role that their pet plays in their lives. To so many clients they are fully fledged members of the family.

The Consultation

I prepare myself and the environment to ensure that there is a quiet atmosphere well before a consultation, and will have some of the macerated oils prepared and a bowl of water ready for the patient. I try to create an ocean of peace so that the animals and their owners are totally relaxed from the minute they walk in through the door.

Over a cup of tea, the owner and I go through a detailed consultation, discussing past history and previous illnesses as well as the diagnosis from the vet. Some animals have been rescued, while others have had a change of owner or suffered challenging behaviour issues; all of these contributory factors make up a picture for me to work with. I offer the client a nice, comfy chair while I squat on a little wooden stool so that I can be at ground level with the animal. My clients are always amused when I start stretching out on the floor so that I can put my hands close to a nervous animal to start the healing. Some animals have experienced trauma in their past and often feel more comfortable lying down under the treatment couch. By end of the session they'll often end up lying happily on the dog bed next to it.

As a holistic animal practitioner, I look at the whole animal and the whole picture, from diet and environment to the effect of stresses going on in the animal's everyday life. Some animals suffer from the effect of pollutants and electromagnetic forces, not to mention the stresses of home life, and it's important to build up a full story before the animal himself gets an opportunity to add his own needs by showing us the oils he selects. I get to see people and animals from all sorts of different environments through home visits to animal sanctuaries both here and abroad, which has widened my understanding of the relationship between humans and animals immeasurably. I see just how important it is to respect where we all come from, and that our roots are the key to understanding who we are.

My aim is to get the body balanced again in order for it to maintain its own health naturally. This concept is known as *homeostasis*, first written about in 1865 by the father of physiology, Claude Bernard. The concept of homeostasis is now routinely taught in veterinary colleges and medical schools. Over the last 50 years, however, the pharmaceutical industry has encouraged conventional medicine to treat symptoms rather than the underlying causes of disease, leaving room for complementary therapists such as me to become 'health detectives' and leave no stone unturned in the search for the whole picture.

Time is the key to understanding how to achieve homeostasis, and I make sure that I spend at least 15 minutes of a consultation with the owner before I start any healing. People are delighted that I ask so many details; they love the opportunity to talk about their animals and I can get a good picture of the relationship just from our preliminary chat. Most of them know instinctively that there are so many factors that can contribute to their pet's condition. After focusing on the presenting illness with their vet, it's often a relief for them to be able to see the bigger picture. Often I'll spend a good deal of time talking to the owner while the animal falls asleep; it's as if he's saying, 'Phew. Someone's listening finally. Now I can relax.' I often find that it is the first time that the client has been listened to.

Melanie and Bud

Sometimes I feel as if I know a client's whole family even if I never meet them. Melanie was one of my very first clients, and taught me so much about the importance of environmental influences. She didn't just bring her tough little jet-black Staffordshire bull terrier Bud to see me, she brought the entire family dynamics into my consulting room.

Melanie had had Bud vaccinated so that the family could take him with them to their holiday home in the south of France, but, following his jabs, he had begun to lose his hair. He had also suffered from diarrhoea, something I see in a lot of dogs who have jabs in order to travel abroad. Bud's behaviour also left a lot to be desired; despite feeling pretty groggy when he arrived in France the last time they had taken him, he had still managed to muster the energy to pick on the neighbour's dog. As none of Melanie's family speaks French, the incident didn't go down well.

I always take my time when introducing animals to oils. They can often elicit a huge emotional release; as mentioned earlier, an animal's sense of smell is far more powerful than ours. When I invited Melanie to offer Bud some oils, I handed them to her very slowly so that Bud had time to focus and decide for himself if he wanted to absorb the aromas or take a lick. One by one, beginning with violet leaf for confidence and then marigold for emotions, I let him select what he needed. He took two drops of marigold, a mild anti-inflammatory and great for any skin condition and hair loss, but completely ignored the neroli and rose.

Melanie is a lovely woman, a classic Liverpudlian with a great sense of humour and a gorgeous smile. She came to that first consultation dressed beautifully in a slim-fitting black leather full-length coat and high-heeled boots, her thick, glossy chestnut hair professionally styled and her beautifully applied make-up all adding up to give the impression of a confident woman in her mid-thirties. Almost immediately, though, I could tell that inside she was desperate to share her feelings with someone. I felt her self-esteem was not quite as bright as her outer self.

Bud, on the other hand, is a rubber ball of a dog, and was bouncing onto the couch and sniffing at everything in the room. Staffies are gorgeous companions and the most affectionate little things, but a couple of centuries ago they were originally bred for fighting and ratting, and their energy, if it's not properly used, can be misinterpreted. I often hear of Staffies being maligned; people associate them with street gangs, yet they make lovely family pets and are extremely loyal. The combination of their physical strength, their weight and their enormous bounding energy, as well as that typical Staffie habit of mouthing or holding your hand in their mouths, can be very off-putting and sometimes frightening if you're not used to dogs. And any animal will pick up on fear. Adrenaline is sweated out through the pores, and dogs' powerful noses will immediately put them on alert. Someone who associates a mouthing Staffie with a biting, fighting dog may find that this impression is made reality by their fearful reaction.

Nevertheless I was surprised when Melanie explained during the consultation how aggressive Bud was with other dogs. She told me how he had been chewing everything in sight, especially the interior of her car as well as her shoes and his own toys. I watched as she kept pulling him back on his chain lead, telling me to be careful of him, warning me that he would tear my chairs up. But Bud was simply desperate to meet me and eager to play. Melanie was misinterpreting her own dog's behaviour.

You often see dogs who are carbon copies of their guardians, but what was interesting was that Melanie and Bud were mirroring each other's behaviour. They were both like coiled springs, which immediately made me wonder what was going on in the family home. I casually asked her a little about her life as I passed an oil to her to give to Bud, and she laughed as she told me that it was a very noisy household. I sensed that she did not find it very funny in reality and encouraged her to talk more about it. She told me that her 17-year-old son and her husband were always shouting at each other – and at her. The two of them always seemed to be letting off steam, and her son's hobbies all seemed to be so loud; he would even let off fireworks in the garden.

I told her that most dogs would be alarmed by this; a dog's hearing is so much more enhanced than ours and it was no surprise that Bud was on edge because of this erratic, chaotic home environment. As Melanie painted the scene, she said that as much as she tried to calm her family down, nobody paid any attention to her. No one seemed to have any respect for her.

Although I love healing animals, I think that one of the most important things that I do is to show their owners that their thoughts, behaviour and feelings have an effect on their pets. When they realize this, and that it can so easily be changed, the focus shifts from pet to owner and allows something quite magical to happen.

We know that animals are much more sensitive to energy than we are. They drink up the emotions of their owners and feel a responsibility to heal their grief and loneliness. It's as if they are an emotional barometer in the home. The moment that owners recognize this is often when they begin to take responsibility for their own feelings and become the leader of the pack that their pets so badly need.

As I crouched down to start the healing, I asked Melanie to relax back and join me in the grounding exercise. I asked her to breathe deeply with me as we tuned in to the healing meditation. As she began to inhale more deeply, her breath became choked and I could tell she was finding it hard to hold the tears back. She tried again but the tears poured down her cheeks. She attempted to stop, apologizing through her sobs, but as I handed her tissues and encouraged her to let it out, she soon sobbed like a child.

I told her how important it is to release anxieties which build up in the body as stress, and, still apologizing, she began to open up. I listened for a long time as she told me about the one-night stand that had changed her life. She had felt so lonely and so under-appreciated at home that the other man's attentions had been too hard to resist. Her husband had always treated her with so little respect that it had rubbed off on her son. They both made her feel stupid, that she owed them all that she had. She regretted her betrayal terribly and had confessed immediately, but both of them had refused to forgive her. She was now even lonelier than she had ever been. The only unconditional love she got was from Bud.

As she told her story, Bud, who had been sleeping quietly, woke up and jumped onto her lap and licked her tears away. I told her that Bud really loved her, that he was her ally – but that made her cry even more. Finally, she agreed to lie on the couch and accept a healing herself while Bud obediently lay under the treatment couch curled up on the dog duvet.

Before falling asleep he looked at me and gave out a satisfied sigh.

After the healing, Melanie told me that although she had a good lifestyle, she had had very little schooling when she was younger and confided in me that she could not read very well. I gave her some pointers about where to find some courses and she left the consulting room that day a very different woman. I heard from her a few months later to say that she felt much more confident, that the literacy course was going well and that Bud's hair loss was a thing of the past. Melanie and Bud are still mirroring each other, but now both of them finally have their feet firmly on the ground.

For Melanie, Bud's skin condition was a catalyst to her finding her way to the healing which changed her life. I believe that that dog was sent to protect Melanie, to be her confidant, but also to help her to realize her potential. She has had a lifetime of allowing men to put her down, to keep her under the thumb. Bud was the first male who could show her what power really meant.

Animals love nothing better than secure boundaries, firm instructions and strong leadership, and this all naturally follows when humans take control of their own lives. There are many avenues towards finding the kind of contentment that comes when chaos has been replaced by clear decision making, but few are as fun or as rewarding as animal healing. The tears that are shed in my clinic are about relief and surrender but also joy as an animal's illness strips back the issues at home. Animals understand that being unhappy makes you – and them – ill, and can physically express their owners' anxieties in ailments such as skin conditions or tumours.

They Are What They Eat

Let food be your medicine and medicine be your food.
HIPPOCRATES

A big part of a consultation is finding out about an animal's food routine. It's an essential part of the jigsaw, and so often it's the key to finding the source of the problem.

A lot of the training I did before I first opened my clinic centred on nutrition, and what I have learnt has changed the way I feed my own animals. Watching animals select the plant oils they need (part of my zoopharmacognosy course) increased my respect for them and I began to look at nutrition in the widest possible sense.

I believe that a well-fed animal is a free animal, in touch with its natural state of being and its sense of purpose. It may be generations since it lived in the wild, but an emotionally well-nourished animal is a powerhouse. Its pride and ego are intact, its will power, energy and enthusiasm have not been compromised. What I see so often in my clinic is the opposite, however: anxiety, fear, worry and domination issues.

When I'm healing an animal I find that most of the imbalances are in the endocrine system, which controls the production of hormones. The digestive centre in particular – the stomach, small intestine, large intestine, spleen and liver (which filters toxins from the body and stores nutrients) – is often where I find the answers.

The pancreatic glands are also in this area, and control insulin and glucagons, which play vital roles in controlling metabolism. The pancreas can't maintain a steady level of glucose, or sugar, in the blood or keep the body supplied with fuel to produce and maintain stores of energy. The amount of diabetes in animals is steadily rising, and this stems from an imbalance in the pancreas. Digestive problems, food allergies, constipation, diabetes, liver complaints, ulcers and stomach tumours are also the kind of ailments that I see all too often. Luckily, most can be treated with a change in diet.

Dried Food
Very often, the way that the body first signals disease is through the skin. I'd go as far as to say that around 80 per cent of my animal patients suffer from flaky or itchy skin or eczema of some kind. Their owners tell me that they think it's something to do with anxiety, and it may well be, but the first question I always ask is 'What do you feed him?' Very often, the answer is the same: dried food. Owners often think that they're doing the best for their animal by following the vet's advice and buying him 'complete' dried food. It's easier, too; they're rushing out to work in the morning and don't want to leave wet food in a bowl on the floor for flies to lay their eggs on or to encourage mice or rats into the house.

I am not against dried food, so long as it is part of a balanced diet including good sources of protein, carbohydrates, minerals, vitamins, fruits and vegetables from natural sources.

Imagine if you were only allowed to eat dried food for the rest of your life. Our bodies are built to enjoy the stimulation of a varied diet; just look at the incisors of an animal. A dog's or cat's are relatively small compared to those of herbivores, whose teeth are designed to grasp and nip off plants and grasses. A dog's canine teeth are well developed to fix and hold their prey and to inflict damage by puncturing deep into the victim's tissues. Its molar and premolar teeth are designed for grinding, and even have raised portions called 'cusps' which help them break up bone and other tough tissues. To limit their diet to a bowl of dried food is enough to make their skin crawl.

At lectures I've been involved in many discussions with vets, and swapped stories about the problems we all see as a result of all-dried-food diets. We've noticed a rise in kidney failure among cats and dogs fed on these foods. The food company reps these days are so slick and vets haven't got time to really look into what they're getting. The science sounds right, but all you need to remember is where these animals come from – that puts it all into perspective.

Hidden Salt and Sugar
I believe that the cheaper pet food manufacturers are contributing to the increase in diabetes in domestic pets by disguising the exact amount of salt and sugar in foods. Sugar has many 'aliases', including:

- maltose
- dextrose
- muscovado (dark brown sugar)
- high-fructose corn syrup
- hydrolysed starch.

Salt, meanwhile, also goes by the name sodium. Given the names these substances hide behind, you would have to be a nutritionist to be able to work out how to feed your pet properly. I see more and more cases of diabetes, obesity and its effects, such as strain on the joints, and much of this comes from excess salt and sugar.

Dogs are carnivores leaning towards omnivores, and they need a balanced diet just like the rest of us. Pet food manufacturers know that wild dogs eat everything from a carcass, and so they use mechanically reclaimed meat including the muscles and bones in their tinned food. They forget that the food wouldn't have been cold from a fridge; a carcass would have been warm and wolfed down within minutes by all members of the pack: a sociable, nutritious family meal.

Many people ask me whether or not the meat they give their dogs should be raw. It takes responsibility to get the balance right, and it is vital that the meat is of the highest quality. Raw or cooked, so much of the cheaper meats are packed with antibiotics due to intensive farming and cramped conditions, where even healthy animals destined for consumption are given antibiotics and growth hormones that are then absorbed by your pet.

My own dogs have cooked chicken and meat and large bones flashed in a hot oven to kill off the high levels of bacteria found on foods that humans have handled. If there are small children around, raw meat on bones is not the most hygienic of things to find left in the back garden. A bone once a month is more than enough for most domestic pets' digestive systems.

I tell my clients that a natural diet for a dog or cat living with human companions is based on *sharing*. Nothing goes to waste in my home: the remains of the chicken carcass goes into a soup or a stock and, once it has been strained, I give it to my dogs, taking care to take out the small, sharp bones. I don't think of leftovers so much as 'set asides', and always cook a little extra at each meal.

Teresa and Heidi

Most pet owners do what they think is best for their animals, sometimes going out of their way to get special treats. I remember when Heidi, a gorgeous Great Dane who was being treated for a dermatological condition by the vet, came to see me. She was the size of a Shetland pony and was losing her hair. Her skin was red-hot, itchy and oozing pus from the raw patches where she had been scratching. The vet had no idea what the source of the problem was, but when we looked more closely at Heidi's diet, her owner Teresa revealed that she was feeding her tripe almost exclusively.

Tripe has been used in the diet of working dogs out in the field from morning to night for years. It's a great source of vital nutrients, but companion dogs exercised once or twice a day simply do not need that level of protein any more. Heidi's organs were reacting in an attempt to process this superfood, and the tripe was being excreted through her skin because her body just couldn't get rid of it any other way. Of course with a body as big as Heidi's, she did need a good source of protein, but chicken was perfectly good enough. I told Teresa that tripe was fine as part of a balanced diet, and within weeks Heidi's new diet had rebalanced her digestive system and her skin condition was a thing of the past.

Let Them Eat Meat

Cats and dogs need meat. I did have a vegetarian dog patient who lived for a very long time, and his owner was dedicated to offering him a very varied natural diet which worked for him. But cats can't exist without meat. They need more protein than dogs, as well as two main nutrients found only in animal tissue: arachidonic acid and taurine. Taurine is an essential amino acid and is found in high quantities in meat and fish, and is practically non-existent in plant-based foods. Mostly, taurine-deficient cats will exhibit signs of depression and shortness of breath, and the deficiency can lead to blindness and, in most cases, death.

In the wild, cats hunt mice, rabbits and small birds; like other carnivores they devour the stomach contents of their prey. They also would eat fruits and nuts, and stolen eggs. Similarly, a dog in the wild would eat everything he could get his paws on. He would kill rabbits and eat absolutely everything on the carcass, including the offal and pre-digested vegetable matter in the stomach of his prey. He would also have eaten berries, nuts, vegetables and fruits. He would also have stolen eggs. My dogs love eggs. When I crack an egg onto an empty saucer, I love the way my gang, especially Morris, licks the white first and then devours the yolk last.

Many people are surprised that I feed oily fish to my own dogs and cat as part of a balanced diet, but it is a very reasonably priced and highly nutritional meal. I suggest it to my cat- and dog-owning clients, because tinned pilchards, sardines and tuna contain Omega 3, 6 and 9, all of which have anti-inflammatory properties. These essential fatty acids (EFAs) are so important in all our diets, and are not only found in sardines but in plant-seed oils like sunflower, olive, calendula and hemp seed. Many animals self-select these for inflammation, pain and joint and cartilage damage, especially elderly pets and those who have broken legs or who have suffered ligament damage earlier in life and are now developing arthritis.

It's always important to introduce new foods slowly, in separate food bowls to monitor how much a dog or cat is taking. With sardines or pilchards, the oil can be discarded at first, then introduced slowly, too.

Max and the Sardines

A tin of sardines is so cheap and yet it's packed with Omega 3 and 6, both of which are great for skin and are anti-inflammatory, so great for keeping joints healthy and in particular for arthritic older animals. I always carry a couple of tins of sardines in my bag just in case I meet an animal who needs them.

On one of my field-study trips abroad, I was working with some vets north of Lisbon and had an opportunity to visit a temple where a Master Lama lived. I am fascinated by the teachings of the Dalai Lama, whose philosophy inspires me to make happiness my goal. Meditation is part of his daily practice, as it is mine, and being in this remote part of Portugal was a great opportunity to find out more about his teachings.

On one free afternoon I headed off by car up a mountain track, driving around hairpin bends and admiring the breathtaking views. Then I came to the gates of a beautiful temple, bedecked with red, golden and yellow brocade. There, at the entry way to some truly stunning gardens, was a beautiful dog, a German shepherd cross-breed with gorgeous, soulful eyes. I went up to him and made a fuss of him, noticing as I ruffled his fur that he had a terrible skin condition. I just stopped short of offering him a tin of sardines, which I always have with me, right there and then.

Two Buddhist monks came to the gate to greet me and I introduced myself and asked if I could meet the Master Lama himself. They agreed and took me to meet him, with Max, the dog, trotting behind us. As the Lama shook my hand, we chatted for a while about the work of the monks, and he showed me into the temple. I felt torn. I really wanted to concentrate on what he was saying to me about the work of his monks here in Portugal, but at the same time my head was racing about the protocol of asking a Master Lama if I could give his dog some sardines for his itching skin. I wondered if he were vegetarian, and whether we were on sacred ground.

I couldn't bear it any longer and asked the Master Lama what he fed his dog. He looked puzzled, but told me that the monks would go to the supermarket and buy supermarket-brand dog food. As reverently as I could, I asked him gently if it was dried food. When he said that it was, I rummaged in my bag for my tin of sardines and asked if I could give it to Max.

I think the Master Lama wrote me off as some kind of English eccentric, but he smiled and said that Max wasn't interested in food. I reminded him that animals are naturally driven by their impulse to eat, and that in the wild Max would be eating wet food that he would hunt for himself. I think the Lama thought of Max as a being of higher consciousness who wasn't interested in the pleasures of the earth. 'You can try,' he told me, still smiling.

Max was wagging his tail and salivating as I opened the ring-pull, and he licked the tin inside out. It didn't need washing before I put it out for recycling. The Lama was very gracious and agreed that he had never seen Max so satisfied.

I spent the day with them and discovered that the lamas' own diet was not much better. Despite their enlightened states, they were all blokes together and, after chatting to them for a while, I suggested that I take them into the kitchen to show them simple ways of cooking. They had shut themselves off from the rest of the world – one of them had even escaped from Tibet – yet they didn't know how to nourish themselves.

As we made our way into the peaceful cool of the temple to meditate together, Max lay outside in the shade, satisfied after his fish lunch. I felt blissful in this beautiful place and thanked Max for introducing me to another side of his world here, and prayed that the lamas would continue to grow in their understanding of how to meet his needs.

As I left, I noticed a harvest display on the table piled high with gorgeous fruits and vegetables and, bang in the middle, a packet of Ritz crackers. I'm a real fruit nut and would have loved something to quench my thirst from the intense heat outside. I willed the Lama to allow me to take some fruit home as he shook my hand and said, 'Thank you so much for what you've done for Max. I want to give you something in return.' I believed that my prayers were about to be answered as he reached into the middle of the harvest display, but instead of fresh fruit, he gave me the box of Ritz crackers!

Local Produce

A lot of what I suggest my clients feed their animals is based on good old-fashioned common sense. Sardines are wonderful for cats and dogs, but they need more than a bit of fish to keep them going. Food from the land rather than from the supermarket is a good start; a perfect diet would include herbs and plants, which animals have been self-selecting for thousands of years, and titbits from the plate just as people have been giving their animal companions since they started living alongside us.

I go to the supermarket to get my basics, but I love going to the butcher and fishmonger or one of my organic farmers down the road. The butcher is not only the best person to talk through how best to feed your family (expert that he is on the cheapest cuts, such as ox heart and liver, and on how to cook them), he's also a dog owner's best friend and will provide all sorts of wonderfully nutritious foods that most of us wouldn't think to give our pets. Tripe is a fabulous food for dogs, but – as Teresa found out with Heidi the Great Dane – it must be eaten in very small quantities. Fresh marrow bones keep teeth clean and are a great source of calcium, and butchers will happily give free bones to their regular customers. A bone a month is plenty for most dogs.

Most people prefer to do one big shop a week because they haven't got time to pop into the local shops. A lot of this is based on the practicalities of juggling a working life with feeding a family, and it may not be possible to store lamb chops bought during your lunch hour at work all afternoon. Increasingly, people are relying on something from the freezer when they get home and giving their pets convenience food, too.

I believe that even the busiest people can change this mindset by buying little and often, and organic as much as possible. As oil prices rise, the price of meat will rise too and higher quality, locally reared and extensively farmed will become a special treat for the weekend. In the meantime, no one can say that a few fresh vegetables from the greengrocer, who also sells pulses and pasta or rice, would be too hard to store at work. Buying for the day also saves money, as there is less waste in the fridge, and most pets will be happy to clear up any remains of the family meal!

Conscious Shopping

If my clients can afford to buy organic, I will insist on it. Apart from the health benefits of organic food, there are enormous environmental advantages, too. Organic farming uses 30 per cent less energy than non-organic farming – and that will become more and more important as the price of oil rises.

Buying organic also means that people tend to think about the bigger issues such as the relationship between low-cost meat and intensive farming methods. They think twice about processed foods and their hidden fats and sugars, and about the link between diet and obesity as well as attention and behavioural problems in children.

It is important to get the question of organic food into perspective. If money is tight, it is much more important to eat plenty of fruit and vegetables – organic or not – than to deprive the family of vital nutrients. And that includes pets. My dogs gnaw on raw broccoli and carrots as if they were bones. It is essential that carrots in particular are organic, because they are taproot vegetables and absorb all the chemicals from fertilizers in the soil.

But food consciousness is rising. Look at Jamie Oliver and Hugh Fearnley-Whittingstall, who are using their positions and influence to expose practices of bad animal husbandry. Most food programmes these days feature local, seasonal produce. As a result, things really are changing. Every single animal deserves our respect and to have the best possible life while it is here on Earth. I would like to see more abattoirs being moved closer to the source of the meat, for example, so that animals do not have to be transported miles in a state of distress.

Once people see their own animal making informed choices about oils, responding to healing and using his spirit to pull himself through serious illness, they are more likely to refuse to buy cheap meat, which they know has come from an intensive background, and to demand better animal husbandry.

A more conscious shopper will opt for organic food both to reduce his own carbon footprint and to encourage more extensive farming so that animals are allowed to root out their own food and self-select what they need, just as they once did. Farmers' markets are allowing farmers to reclaim their power over their production, and climate change is forcing us into a more balanced relationship with our environment.

Mother Nature, the real top of the food chain, is taking control and throwing us back into instinctive living. That's evidence to me that consciousness is shifting and vibrations are rising. But don't be too surprised if we humans hasten our own destruction and it's the animals who inherit the Earth.

Shaun, Christine and Frosty

Food is also really important in supporting an animal being treated for serious disease. Shaun and Christine brought their lovely little six-year-old West Highland terrier, Frosty, to me after their vet had diagnosed the swelling under her armpits, on her stomach and between her legs as cancerous. Although swellings like this can often be a simple build-up of fluid in the lymph glands (which are designed to deal with the body's waste), a biopsy of the lymph nodes and an ultrasound scan of Frosty's stomach had confirmed that she was living with one of the most aggressive forms of lymph cancer. With chemotherapy she was given six months at the outside; without it, just two weeks. Shaun and Christine had also been told that her breathing would deteriorate quickly if they did not act immediately, so they had taken her straight to the Veterinarian Referrals Cancer and Critical Care Centre in Laindon, Essex, reputedly the best animal cancer treatment facility in Europe. Scan results showed that, although the cancer hadn't spread to Frosty's vital organs, the oncologist was concerned about a large tumour in her spleen. Frosty would have to have chemotherapy every Friday for the next six weeks, after which time her condition would be reassessed. They were sent away with a two-week course of antibiotics and steroids.

Veterinary hospitals do amazing work with animals, but the problem with conventional medicine is always the same: no one asks about diet and lifestyle. Shaun and Christine, like me, believe that you have to look at health holistically if you want real results.

When they brought Frosty in to see me, it soon emerged that there were plenty of deep-rooted issues going on which may well have contributed to her stress and given the cancer the power to grow. Christine and Shaun told me that Frosty had always been a stressed dog, hiding behind their other dog, Angel. Some animals worry more than others and, as a breed, the West Highland terrier is an anxious one. They can suffer tremendously from stress, and many have skin problems and stomach complaints.

Animals also reflect the emotions of their owners, and if Frosty were a person she would be a silent worrier, just like Christine. Christine cares passionately about everyone else and, although she is a very grounded person, she thinks too much for her own good. Frosty empathizes with her; if she could put a paw on her arm, she would.

We know that disease is caused by a myriad of contributing factors, and when Shaun and Christine first told me about Frosty's cancer, their intention was clear from the first session: they weren't going to hand over the responsibility to the healer. They were absolutely part of it from the beginning.

Shaun has strong healing abilities himself; his mother is a healer, too, and he knew how important it was to include the whole family if they were to heal Frosty.

Angel, Frosty's dog companion, came along too. Although not her biological sister, Angel and Frosty are devoted to each other, with Angel taking the lead in the relationship. Frosty is a timid little dog and very much in her shadow. I quickly picked up that Angel was terribly worried about Frosty, and we all recognized that she would also need support during this difficult time.

As I settled down with both dogs in the clinic to offer the oils, Frosty showed a particular interest in my macerated calendula oil. I poured some onto a plastic tray and she gently licked it up. Calendula is well known for its natural anti-inflammatory properties. Frosty then selected the carrot seed, a blood tonic and anti-coagulant. This made me wonder if her chemotherapy treatment was affecting her platelets (the body's normal clotting agent).

As for diet, the relationship between food and antioxidants is essential in helping chemotherapy fight the spread of the cancer. Frosty, however, had always been fed conventional dog food. Good food is necessary to support the body as it deals with the side effects of steroids and antibiotics, not to mention the chemo and all the emotional stress involved in travelling to and from hospital. Vets are unanimous these days about keeping steroids on a short course because of the long-term health implications. They understand that steroids can suppress the immune system if used long term.

When I explained about the need to give Frosty organic meat and vegetables to support her through the stress of this kind of intervention, Shaun and Christine immediately set about writing a shopping list. Some of it is not quite what they expected, but Frosty loves her new diet: avocados, kiwis, bananas, fish and blueberries (which are so high in vitamin C that they were ranked top for antioxidant activity among 40 fruits and vegetables, in research done at Tufts University in Boston). Breakfast these days usually consists of eggs, tuna, prawns or pilchards laced with garlic and sprinkled with ground walnuts, almonds and pumpkin seeds. Evening meals are usually minced beef or lamb, liver, kidney or chicken – all organic, of course – with tomatoes, spinach, grated carrots and a crushed clove of garlic. In between meals, she gets a bowl of fruit: watermelon is a favourite as it cleanses the lymph glands, with blueberries and bananas (a good source of potassium). Even pineapples, kiwi fruit and strawberries go down well.

Manuka honey has become a regular bedtime treat after Frosty self-selects the calendula oil from Christine's hand, as among its other valuable properties it helps to boost blood levels. Salmon is a favourite, as is most seafood, apart from smoked mackerel which Frosty refuses to eat. Shaun and Christine were astonished when I told them that she would have recognized this as a processed product.

Christine already knew that natural yoghurt can help keep the good gut flora alive while taking antibiotics, but she didn't think it would work on a dog. I use Yeo Valley yoghurt and recommend it to all my patients. My mum lives near the Yeo Valley farm, and I've been very impressed with the people and philosophy behind it. Energetically, it matters how food is produced, even down to the way the business side of things is handled. Frosty gobbled it up.

Nutritionists and oncologists recommend foods containing lysopene (also known as lycopene), which neutralizes aggressive free-radicals. It's easily found: tomatoes are packed with it – cooked and raw. It's even found in ketchup. Frosty gets hers from watermelon, where it's really abundant.

Beta carotene, found in carrots, is another must, but the carrots have to be organic; if not, the chemicals in the pesticides cancel out any real healing benefits.

Unfortunately, broccoli – which is so rich in beta carotene, folate and potassium as well as vitamin C, sulphoraphane and indols, which are known to prevent cancer – has a bit of an adverse effect on Frosty's digestive system: a fact she demonstrates with silent but deadly reminders during our healing sessions as she drifts off into a relaxing snooze...

Frosty doesn't just self-select when she's in the clinic; when she's out in my garden playing with my terriers before a session, she wolfs down the pansies, and Christine says that she loves sniffing the pine trees in her own garden at home. There's obviously something in there that she needs and, whatever it is, it must be good for her; her vets can't get over the fact that she is not being sick or feeling nauseous and that she hasn't suffered any side effects from chemotherapy.

The behaviour of both Frosty and Angel has changed enormously over the course of our healing sessions. Initially

Angel had been a little jealous of the attention Frosty was getting, so I would always ask them who wanted to come first, and Angel would always confirm her place in the pack by coming forward. Slowly, over the months, Angel has given space for Frosty to get what she needs. Shaun and Christine tell me that neither dog has ever been the kind to sit on their laps, but during the healing sessions Angel sits on Shaun's lap while I heal Frosty. Shaun naturally follows my lead as I ground all of us before starting the healing, and he copies my hand movements on Angel. It's wonderful for me to know that everyone in the room is attuned. That kind of synergy is a rare gift for us all.

It isn't just the dogs' behaviour that is shifting. Christine, once such a shy woman next to the charismatic and charming Shaun, is becoming more self-confident by the day. The dogs love her mum so much and she can feel it. While Shaun is focusing on Angel, I have been encouraging Christine to become more involved in the healing, too. It's clear that Shaun knows what to do, but there is something special about Christine, too, and I want her to know that. I encourage her to look at the tumours and send her focus to Frosty's stomach and spleen, to focus on shrinking them in her mind's eye, gradually making them smaller and smaller, then imagining tying a knot to cut off the blood supply to the cancerous cells. Our intention is for Frosty's body to become well once again. In one session, both Christine and I found ourselves focusing on the left lymph gland, and I wasn't surprised to find out later (as borne out by hospital tests) that the cancer there was more aggressive than in the right gland.

As the healings began to settle Frosty, Shaun and Christine have watched with amazement at how assertive and how brave she has become, not just with the way that she is dealing with treatment but also with Angel. In return, Angel has become less stressed, too. No one likes to be out in front, or to be depended upon, all the time. Now when they are out on walks, Frosty, who had always stuck to Christine's side, is now exploring with Angel, who is thrilled to have a proper playmate.

So many of my clients think that because their dog has cancer they have to wrap them in cotton wool for the rest of their time together, but life doesn't come to a halt for a dog who is ill. Frosty needs the endorphins produced by the joy of chasing a squirrel back up a tree or a rabbit back into its warren. It makes her feel good.

I am still healing Frosty and am on the end of the phone for her lovely owners whenever they need me. Shaun called me recently to tell me that her red blood count was down. She had become almost anaemic, so much so that they couldn't give her the chemo. I suggested giving her some liver to raise her iron intake, as it is a great source of iron if fed as part of a mixed diet. It worked a treat. A week of small doses was enough to raise her red blood count. As with tripe, it's important to limit the intake of such an iron-rich food, and I have seen it oozing out of dogs' skin when they are fed it exclusively, because the organs are working overtime to digest it and the sebaceous glands are called upon to excrete it. A wolf in the wild may eat the heart, liver and other intestines because of their high nutritional value, but domestic dogs just can't handle too much offal without the exercise to burn all that energy off.

Frosty's cancer is now in remission, although after the eighth dose of chemotherapy she developed a bladder inflammation, a direct side effect of the drugs, which meant that she became incontinent. A twice-daily belly rub with a compound of aloe vera and yarrow is giving her relief, but it is not just the chemo that is causing the problems. As a result of the first course of steroids she has put on a lot of weight, which has put more pressure on her vital organs and spine. A recurrence of a previous vertebrae problem would mean no exercise for several weeks and a vicious circle of trying to control her weight, so we are all working together to ensure that we manage each of these issues.

When she comes to see me, she marches into the consultation room and is ready for the healing. She seems to be so grateful to us all for everything that we're doing, for this dedication. Shaun and Christine make a round trip of 200 miles for their dog, but they believe it's worth it. Seeing Frosty so full of life vindicates their decision to treat her cancer holistically. They doubt whether she would have made it beyond those first couple of months without the healings and change of diet.

As we go to press, the vets have given her the all-clear, and they cannot give a medical explanation as to why the lymph sarcomas in the spleen have shrunk so dramatically. Frosty's story is about hope, about the astonishing power of healer, owner and animal coming together for the highest intentions. Animals are living so much longer these days, and as their human owners' consciousness rises, the most phenomenal experiences can change not only their animals' life expectancy, but the quality of life of those around them.

Allergies and Food Intolerance

Food allergies are as common in pets as they are in humans, and can be a significant cause of a wide range of symptoms in animals. Vets estimate that 15 per cent of all allergic skin disease in dogs and cats may be caused by food hypersensitivity; it may be the second most common cause of pruritis (itchy skin) in cats and the third most common cause in dogs. There does not appear to be any sex or breed predisposition, although I do see a lot of German shepherds, West Highland terriers and Labrador retrievers who seem to have a high incidence of food allergies.

Food allergies affect the skin and can bring on itching and hair loss as well as redness and inflammation, but they can also affect the gastrointestinal system and the nervous system. Gastrointestinal signs include vomiting, diarrhoea, sometimes bloody diarrhoea and straining and increased frequency of bowel movements. I've even seen animals suffering seizures which have been associated with food hypersensitivity. Hyperactivity, depression, irritability, arthritis and joint pain, asthma, chronic bronchitis, hypoglycaemia and sinusitis, I've seen it all.

It's vital to check these symptoms with the vet first, but figuring it out can often call for a bit of simple detective work. Check when the itching or other symptoms began to show up. Have the washing powder and fabric conditioner for his bedding been changed recently? What about his food? If the symptoms stop when the old powder and food are replaced, the detective work is often done.

Food trials are the easiest way of figuring out food allergies, for both humans and animals. I usually recommend an elimination diet as the first step when diagnosing food allergies. This means limiting your pet to one protein source and one carbohydrate source that he hasn't tried before. For instance, if he was on a basic dog or cat food with wheat and cereal and beef as its main ingredients, I'd suggest a home-made diet of fish and rice, which has a higher ratio of protein, or one of the hypoallergenic diets of prepared fish and rice.

It can take many months to see a change; some food elimination trials have found that symptoms did not improve for six months. I usually see improvements within a fortnight. Once we have worked out that the animal patient is sensitive to a particular pet food, we can then work out which foods are causing the reaction. Is it the carbohydrate source such as wheat or cereal, or the protein source such as beef, chicken or fish? Could it be something else: flavours, preservatives, artificial colours? All of these are possible and we can try a food provocation trial next, in which the wheat is reintroduced to see if the symptoms recur.

The most common food allergens for pets include beef, chicken, pork, wheat, corn, soybeans, eggs and dairy products, particularly the cheap cuts of meat and dairy which are packed with antibiotics and can suppress the immune system. I always tell owners that if they use branded pet foods, they should experiment by changing over to another, keeping note of all the different foods and chemicals that are in the pet food.

Some people choose to cook a home-made diet for their pet, which makes it easier to keep track of the list of ingredients. Certain toys and snacks such as bones or other processed chews may have offending substances in them as well, and therefore need to be removed during food elimination trials.

There are blood tests for food allergies, but there is still some controversy about how reliable they are. Food sensitivities can also mimic other sensitivities such as inhalant or contact allergies, flea allergies as well as parasitic infections.

Nature's larder is also a fabulous medicine cabinet: garlic is a natural antibiotic and kills internal parasites as the smell passes through the skin to become a natural flea repellent.

Many owners of rabbits and small furries such as guinea pigs feed their pets exclusively on dried food, but these pets are herbivores and need grass. Their teeth are especially designed with flat surfaces that break their food to pulp and make tough cellulose-based structures like grass easier to digest. Herbivores' teeth grow throughout their lives to replace the surfaces as they get ground down, and herbivores have to eat for a significantly greater portion of each day to obtain the energy that they need – something to remember when keeping a house rabbit indoors all day. I've seen the fluorescent colour of rabbits' urine after being fed a diet of additives – it's not pretty!

Tony and Tricia

Often I need to see a client at home to understand properly what is going on with a pet. Mostly a consultation will tell me what I need to know, but I always welcome the opportunity to have a look at the home environment – and I usually head straight for the fridge! Most of the answers can be found here, and owners are usually only too eager to make whatever changes are needed for the sake of their beloved pet.

When Tony asked me to come and see his late wife's guinea pig, Tricia, he thought that I would simply be treating the lymphomas that were all over Tricia's body. He didn't realize that a Gillian McKeith would be coming his way to change both his and his guinea pig's life.

Tony is an attractive, slim gentleman in his early 50s. His wife Marilyn had died from cancer a year before I met him and he was still grieving terribly. His wife had begged him to look after her beloved guinea pig and, although he was struggling, he had kept his promise. He showed me a picture of Marilyn, and I noticed that she looked remarkably similar to Tricia, the guinea pig. They do say that pets often have something about them that resembles their owners, but these two both sported a luscious head of wavy, jet-black hair.

Tricia sniffed me as I chatted to Tony to get a feel for how she spent her days, what she was eating, how much fresh air she was getting. He told me that she lived inside all the time because he was frightened of her being taken by the foxes that use his garden as a pathway to the woods behind his house. He told me that they would watch telly together in the evening, Tricia on a hand-embroidered cushion stitched by Marilyn, perched on Tony's chair, nibbling on a carrot, and Tony tucking into a bar of something nice. He said he found solace in her company; Tricia was Tony's life now that Marilyn was gone, and I quickly realized that he was so worried about losing her that he was compromising her quality of life by trying to keeping her safe.

As we talked I began to put my hands around Tricia's body without directly touching her, and I sensed Tony's anxiety. He didn't just seem sad; his sense of fear was palpable. Tricia was lapping up the healing so I stayed on the floor with her and continued chatting gently with Tony. He seemed terribly lonely as I asked him a little about his life. He told me that since Marilyn had died, he had found it difficult to find the motivation to go out much. Then he quickly clammed up and brought our attention back to Tricia, who was sniffing around my knees again.

I asked him about Tricia's diet and explained the relationship between food and cancer, and wellbeing in general. I made sure that Tony recognized that this applied to every living being; it hadn't escaped my attention that Tony had not been feeding himself properly either. Food was not high on his list of priorities, it seemed.

Tricia needed to eat grass; that much was clear. Her genes had come all the way from the plains of Argentina and Peru to a pretty terraced house in Somerset. I told him that she should eat good-quality guinea-pig mix and a regular supply of good-quality meadow hay. But she also needed cancer-blasting food like tomatoes and red peppers, which have high levels of beta carotene and contain lycopene, the big buzz word in oncology at the moment. Fruits and vegetables also contain vitamin C, an antioxidant which science knows to be an essential cancer-buster and which guinea pigs must be given every day, as they haven't got the enzyme that manufactures or stores this essential vitamin. It's found in parsley, kale leaves, broccoli stems, dandelion leaves, cabbage, spinach, peas, grapes, kiwi and oranges, yet so often guinea pigs are fed a dried diet of pellets packed with chemicals. I have been saying for a long time that I believe that the high incidence of guinea-pig cancer is due to a lack of vitamin C in their diets. I see many so many of these little pets suffering from lethargy and enlarged, stiff joints, rough coats, eye and nose discharge, and I believe that it could all be avoided with a little fresh fruit and veg.

We looked in Tony's fridge to see what fresh vegetables he had, and we chucked away the junk food stacked on the shelves. So often, men don't look after themselves well if their partner is no longer sharing the home. But Tricia's health was the most important thing in the world to Tony, and he was determined to right the wrongs that might have contributed to her disease.

I asked Tony to start shopping at the organic section in his local supermarket, or, better still, support his farmers and bring down the food miles by buying locally.

He was still adamant that it was not safe for Tricia to be in the garden. I asked him if Marilyn had let her run around outside and he sheepishly admitted that she would be horrified to find her living indoors. But he just couldn't risk it; Tricia was all he had now and he had promised Marilyn that he would look after her. I told him that he would just have to bring the outside inside and place plastic trays of turf in an area of the sitting room.

We arranged another session, and I helped him put the turf down. I wanted to show Tony that, even with cancer, a good diet and an improved mental attitude could vastly improve Tricia's quality of life – and his. Despite the cancer, Tricia seemed fairly well; as we laid the turf she ran around between us, obviously loving the fact that we were on her level, and we chatted about an eating plan for the two of them. I asked Tony to keep a food diary for me so we could have regular updates as he adjusted to his new diet. I wanted to create a diet that would raise his self-esteem and enable him to feel fitter, to live the life that he really should be leading.

Tricia was happy now and, as I began to put my hands out for a healing, I noticed Tony's interest. He told me later that he had never heard of healings before, but it was the first time that he had seen such a brightness in Tricia's eyes for a very long time. Gently, I suggested that I could do some healing on him, too. Disease, I explained, is hard on everyone. Tentatively he agreed.

I always take my mobile treatment couch with me in the car for these kinds of occasions, and he settled down and closed his eyes. I took him through the attunement process and suggested that he imagine a hotel in his mind's eye with a number of different rooms off a central corridor. I asked him to describe the surroundings, and as he told me about the stunning backdrop of a quiet forest studded with bluebells, I asked him to go into the hotel and into the first room he saw, quietly closing the door behind him. There he would see someone he needed to talk to. He told me in a tiny voice that Marilyn was there. I asked him to have the conversation that he needed to have with her, then to come out of the room and carefully close the door, locking it behind him.

In other rooms he found other members of his family, including his father who had also died of cancer, and again, he was able to have the conversation with him that he needed to have. In this safe environment of a meditation, he met friends whom he had loved and lost as he'd closed himself off from the outside world. I assured him that he could go back into the hotel any time he liked, either in a guided meditation with me, or, with practice and maybe with a meditation CD, on his own. Afterwards, he sobbed, and the grief of losing his wife finally found an outlet and began to dissolve.

After the session in the imaginary hotel, Tony began to talk about his wife openly, telling me how frightened he had been. Her death had left him feeling so alone, and he had never let anyone close since. He confessed that he was frightened of getting close to anyone, and that now his whole life revolved around Marilyn's guinea pig. He wouldn't even go on holiday because of Tricia.

Together, we worked on a plan for the time they still had together, and vowed to change the way they both ate so that they would be able to live a more active life while they still had it. The more he let go of his fear of losing Marilyn, the more confident he felt about letting Tricia into the garden to graze on real grass and to feel the earth under her feet.

Despite the prognosis two years ago, Tricia is still with us, although she now lives outside in the day and spends her evenings inside, cuddled up on her hand-embroidered cushion with both of them tucking into organic carrot crudités in front of the telly. Her grassy turf from B&Q has been placed on the compost heap where it belongs. Tony has released himself from the stranglehold of fear, and is dating a lovely woman he met through a mutual friend. If I didn't know better, I'd swear that last time I was over I saw Tricia smiling.

Joan, Simon and Mimi

Of course it wasn't appropriate to have a guinea pig indoors, but it took the process of doing it for Tony to release his fears and finally to let Tricia out into the garden. Many cat owners, however, don't have the luxury or feel that they can let their cats run free. I know that lots of people live where it's difficult to let their cats out and they have to work with what they've got. Cats do get run over on busy roads, but I see many rescue cats who have lived naturally in their former homes and who are then kept inside as house cats and I feel their sadness. They have tasted a freedom that they no longer have access to and they feel deeply traumatized.

I had a phone call a couple of years ago from a Scottish lady called Joan, who told me that she just couldn't get her cat out from under the bed. She knew that Mimi was ill with stomach cancer but there was nothing she could do to tempt her out. Animals don't usually let life come to a halt just because they are ill, so Mimi's behaviour had to be a response to something else.

When I got to the house, the first thing I noticed was how dark it was. All the curtains were closed and the atmosphere was heavy throughout the house. Joan and her husband Simon were pretty withdrawn, too, and when they closed that door behind me, it felt that we were closing ourselves off from the outside. I wondered what could have happened to them to make them so afraid of the world.

We sat down to do the initial consultation to see if there were any obvious causes as to why Mimi was being so stubborn. There was nothing obvious from the cat's physical history so I asked a little more about their lifestyle. Joan told me that she worked for a very small company as an administrator, but it was clear to me that she disliked her job. She told me how she had come from Scotland to be with Simon after meeting him on the internet and intuitively I felt that she might have left unfinished business back at home.

Joan seemed to me to be a very frustrated person who poured much of her energy into her cat. She was her baby. When I found out that Mimi was a rescue cat and her previous owner had allowed her outside, I realized what was going on. Joan was so frightened that she would never come back that she refused to let her out at all. Mimi was manifesting all her fear of the outside world by hiding away under the bed.

Simon had been suffering from depression on and off since a teenager and told me that as a result, their life was very quiet, that they didn't have any friends at all. They kept the curtains shut all day to keep the world out, and would even go to Tesco at night to avoid meeting anyone. I wondered if the cat was picking up on this and hiding herself away, too.

After my consultation, I went into the bedroom and lay down on the floor. I began to focus my attention on creating a relaxed, peaceful, positive atmosphere. I encouraged Joan and Simon to join me in the healing so that they would know how to continue themselves after I had gone. I asked them to focus on their breathing. As we gently breathed in and out, we focused on expanding the diaphragm and on the out-breath, gently letting it go, as if it were a balloon deflating.

This basic act of meditation slows down the mind and the breathing. It's important not to let thoughts pop up; detaching from such distractions when healing means that you can focus on creating positive thoughts and feelings of your animal being healed. Healers call this 'positive intention'. With these loving thoughts, the healer gains an inner feeling of strength and confidence and is able to share this with their animals.

It really helps to use guided visualization to keep the mind focused and so I asked Joan and Simon on the next out-breath to visualize the breath travelling down into their legs and feet and to feel the carpet beneath them. I then asked them to visualize a beautiful day with the sun shining and to imagine feeling the warmth of the sun's rays on their faces. I could see that they were responding to this well so I asked them to include Mimi in this vision, and to share these loving feelings with her. These creative visualization techniques can help to induce a very relaxed, happy and calm state from which to start the healing session. Simon said that he had never felt so relaxed.

There was a beautiful calmness in the room and although it was quite dark, I could just see Mimi under the bed peering out at me with her huge eyes. She meowed, as if she was saying, 'Hello.' She gingerly moved towards me, seemingly curious to meet me. I held out my hand as she sniffed and rubbed her head in my fingers and I felt I had her permission to continue the healing session. Wave after wave of positive unconditional love travelled between Mimi and me, and she came out from under the bed, arching her neck and back and purring. I wasn't asking anything more than she was prepared to give. There were no strings attached and she knew it.

I had the very strong feeling that Joan wanted so much to be loved that she was demanding too much from her. She was suffocating Mimi. It's so important to give anyone, animals included, enough space for a relationship to find its own way, and to give love unconditionally.

After half of an hour of the healing, I completed the session by giving thanks and we watched as Mimi walked out from under the bed towards Joan and Simon. Joan's reaction was fascinating. Although she was pleased, I could also see some resentment in her face. She had told me that the cat would simply not come out, and although she had invited me in, there was something very confronting for her about watching this change.

I asked her to consider letting Mimi outside. Ironically, they had a lovely little back garden that Simon tended with great care, but neither of them would let the cat into it. I suggested that they buy a cat lead so that Mimi couldn't run away when she went outside, but when I went back the third time, although they had bought one, they still were too afraid to use it.

Eventually I persuaded them to open the back door. Of course Mimi didn't want to go out at first. You could see her thinking, 'Wow, what's that?' but when she took her first step out, the look on her face was priceless. She put her nose in the air and stood, head back, taking in the air. As she lifted her paws high with each step and planted them gently on the soft grass, it was like she was walking on the moon. She took in the beautiful scent of the red rose bush in the middle of the little garden and then, very slowly, walked to each corner, sniffing, head held high and gently planting her feet on the luscious grass. We spent about half an hour with her on the lead, just allowing her to smell everything. It was beautiful to watch.

I knew that it would take time for them to let Mimi wander freely in the garden and so I asked them to bring some of the outside inside. Scratching posts can be made out of large broken branches straight out of the woods. Synthetic scratching posts with play things are fine but I am concerned about the chemicals in them and if the natural option is on the doorstep, why not use it? Cats love to roll in grass, which can be grown in trays and placed somewhere like a utility room. Catnip is a luxury for cats, as we saw with Shauny, and is also easy to grow. Aloe vera plants are fine and cats may self-select and nibble the leaves. Again, these grow happily in pots. Keeping the environment as natural as possible means limiting chemicals, so go easy on the fragrances. Cats smell of cats. Sensitivities and respiratory problems so often arise from domestic products that are packed with chemicals, from carpet cleaners to washing liquids.

I could tell that Simon and Joan wanted to talk. Simon's hands were shaking as he made me a cup of tea. I congratulated him on his beautiful garden and gradually got him talking. I felt that he was terribly lonely and so I gently suggested that he hire himself out to people in the area as a gardener in his spare time. His face lit up. He could see that maybe there was life outside that house for him.

When I rang to check up on them a year and a half later, Mimi had just died of the stomach cancer. They had buried her under that beautiful red rose bush and I was so pleased that her resting place had been in the great outdoors.

Simon had started doing odd jobs in local gardens and he sounded so much brighter, his voice full of something that felt like hope. Maybe it will be a longer road for Joan, but it was she who first called me in, who read an article about the animal healer who heals their guardians too. Maybe it won't be so long before she draws those curtains and lets the sunshine in again.

Healing animals can often be the beginning of change, but I'm not always around to see the conclusion. Sometimes the best I can do is to turn a light on in a dark area and show the owner where the issues behind her animal's problem really lie. Then I leave it to the animals to continue to shine that light.

Alex and Sacha

Sometimes vets just do not have the time to play detective in the way that I can. Often, my clients take a suggestion from my clinic to the vet for confirmation, so that a carefully planned package of veterinary care, healing and support can then be worked out between us. This is what happened with Alex and Sacha.

I first met Alex and her gorgeous Samoyed, Sacha, years ago when I was out walking my Jack Russell, Alf, and my boxer, Bruce. Samoyeds are such beautiful dogs and were originally used by the Sami tribe of Siberia to herd reindeer. They are a fantastically tough breed with a double-layered coat to help them survive in the harsh tundra, but are wonderfully good-natured and loyal.

Alf and Bruce vied for Sacha's attention and she flirted with both of them over many walks together, and we all became good friends. One day while we were out walking, Alex showed me a skin problem Sacha had developed on her left ear. The vet had given her antibiotics, antihistamines and steroids, but the condition had worsened and developed into a haematoma on the ear. I told Alex that I had successfully treated a similar problem that Alf had developed after colliding with another dog while playing.

Vets do not always like to take radical action straight away with ear haematomas; popping them can often cause a secondary infection and so vets prefer to make the animal comfortable first with antibiotics and anti-inflammatories. After examining Alf, my vet was more than happy for me to treat this myself with a mix of my fresh aloe vera liquidized with fresh garlic and a few drops of yarrow applied to the outside of his hot, swollen ear morning and night. After a month of treatment, it had disappeared completely.

The vet had respected my supportive role as a healer, but as Sacha was on medication, I would have to rely on hands-on healing for now. I asked Alex to bring her over, and after several healings at the clinic and the healing meditation evenings, the haematoma on her ear did indeed clear up. But the problem quickly moved to her bottom and Sacha insisted on chewing at it incessantly. Alex checked with the vet, and he agreed that I could soothe the scabs with a cooling topical application of aloe vera, yarrow and peppermint on her tail. I could see that this gave her immediate relief, but I was racking my brain about the root cause of this condition.

The vet was conducting various tests for parasites and bacterial and fungal infections, but even though they were all negative, he prescribed such a cocktail of allopathic medicine that I could only observe Sacha rather than participate. I found this incredibly frustrating. I like to see what is working or not. It's no good just treating the symptoms without establishing the cause, and so far all the tests had proved inconclusive. The vet really didn't know what to do next; Sacha was given a buster collar, described as an unusual presentation and told to come back regularly for check-ups.

Alex was terribly upset. She would come for healings both for herself and for Sacha after a visit to the vet just to calm herself down. I kept the vet informed of my progress, especially as we began to see if the macerated oils would make a difference. As she sniffed the oils, Sacha was far more decisive than the vet had been and went mad for macerated calendula oil, an anti-inflammatory, antiseptic and antifungal for stressed or fretful animals. It also contains vitamin A, which is rich in sulphur and an excellent blood cleanser with antifungal action. She also self-selected seaweed absolute, an incredibly thick liquid extract from the bladderwrack family and an electrolyte for balancing body fluids. With her hot coat for the Siberian tundra, it was possible she needed something to balance the vital salts needed at the adrenals.

While I was healing Sacha, I noticed how much I was drawn to certain endocrine glands, especially the adrenals and the pancreatic glands. Sacha was ushering me towards her stomach and flanks with her head and would then sink deeper into a relaxed state with a sigh. I couldn't tell what was causing her condition, but it seemed that she knew that it was coming from her stomach area. I suggested that she had more tests to see if she had developed any sensitivity to pathogens such as pollen or insects or even food.

Sure enough, the blood tests showed an intolerance to white fish, wheat, soya, house dust mites, and even a number of trees and meadow grasses native only in the UK. We changed her diet to a fantastic brand of wet food called Natures Menu and Naturediet which includes varieties such as lamb, cooked brown rice, peas and carrots, and chicken and vegetables. Alex topped up Sacha's diet with fresh chicken and mince. She also stopped taking Sacha for country walks, choosing instead a park where the grass was very short and a good distance away from the trees.

I continued making up soothing lotions based on fresh aloe vera and yarrow, and Sacha continued to choose the calendula macerated oil. She loved the healing sessions and would lie over my knees with her underbelly resting on top of my thighs, insisting that I heal her flanks and undercarriage.

Eventually she would relax and I would feel the tension leave her body as she sighed in relief. The pancreas (the production site for insulin) is situated in the stomach and, when faulty, it can't produce enough insulin for the body to store glucose, carbohydrates, fats or proteins, which affects all the other major endocrine glands.

I was concerned that with so much of an imbalance of adrenal and pancreatic energy pulsating through my hands, it would have a chain reaction and cause metabolic chaos, putting an enormous strain on Sacha's body. I suggested that Alex have her tested for diabetes, as her hormones felt totally out of balance. She hadn't presented typical symptoms of diabetes such as increased thirst and urination, but I couldn't dismiss the fact that every time I conducted a healing, I felt that the adrenals were in overdrive and out of synch with the rest of Sacha's body.

Poor old Sacha was on and off the steroids, and both the vet and Alex were aware of the implications on her immune system. When she got sick, she needed a course of antibiotics and an x-ray and we were back to square one. The vet was baffled by why Sacha wasn't responding to treatment and, probably as a last resort, he finally agreed to test her for diabetes. It came back positive.

Diabetes is a very serious condition and must not be treated at home without seeing the vet. Natural remedies can only support allopathic medicine, but a low-sugar diet is vital, with set meals of fixed volume to stabilize insulin levels in the body. It's important to be very strict with ingredients, to keep meals simple and to inform other members of the household of the new routine. Stress can aggravate symptoms, so the more the whole family knows about the condition, the better.

Because Sacha had sensitivities to certain foods, I suggested to Alex that she very slowly and, with very small amounts, increase Sacha's fruit intake (as the soluble fibre helps to control blood-sugar levels). Sacha loved the bananas and nectarines. Most fruits and vegetables are alkaline-forming, which helps to retain bone density, while also being rich in vitamin C, which helps with the absorption of the important minerals calcium and magnesium. This is critical when the immune system is as impaired as Sacha's was.

I also suggested that Alex offered her a small amount of nuts on a separate plate from her other food. Most fresh unsalted nuts, such as almonds, brazils, cashews and hazelnuts, are an excellent source of vitamin E – an antioxidant – a good skin conditioner and high in magnesium, which the body uses to maintain energy. Vitamin E also supports the thyroid gland, which plays a major part in metabolic action in the body, a major worry with animals with diabetes, who can experience sharp weight gain or loss. I suggested to Alex that she use a pestle and mortar to grind the nuts up so that they wouldn't simply come out the other end undigested and unabsorbed, as can often happen when dogs wolf down their dinner.

But Sacha was deteriorating badly after the steroids, and it was touch and go as to whether or not she would make it. She wouldn't eat at all, and as insulin can't be given without food, this was causing yet another complication. Her blood-glucose level should have been between 5 and 12, but was an astonishing 47.

The vet had already started talking to Alex about putting Sacha to sleep, but Alex and Sacha refused to give up and I promised to support them both in any way I could. She did begin to eat again after another healing, but, perhaps more amazingly, her glucose levels plummeted to 25 after the first session, and decreased even further with subsequent healings. This was evidence of how homeostasis, the natural balance of the body, can be achieved though healing. Alex was thrilled; Sacha was now able to have insulin injections twice a day after eating.

It seemed diabetes had been the main cause of her skin problems and once she was on insulin, most of the scabs quickly disappeared. Her hair grew back and she put on weight. It had taken the vet seven months to diagnose her diabetes, but her blood glucose was now down to 10, a perfectly acceptable level.

The following year, however, Sacha began to develop arthritis and, despite the healings, she had to be given morphine, which made her blood-glucose level shoot up again. Her skin problems flared up as a result and the vet even suggested removing the end of her tail if she could not stop chewing it. Again, Alex came to me and asked for help and I made up my aloe vera topical application and Alex applied it regularly. After a week, it was enough to save Sacha's tail.

Sacha was still self-selecting the anti-inflammatory yarrow and calendula macerated oils and enjoying the healings. Even though the vet had raised the euthanasia issue again, Alex knew that Sacha was a survivor; her Sami ancestry had made her as tough as old boots But this journey over the past two years had brought them so much closer together and, even though she was beginning to lose weight now, Alex believed in her gorgeous dog's inner strength and admired her so much for it. She might have been physically weakening, but she was still utterly engaged in her life, enjoying her walks and loving the healings.

When the time came, Alex knew that she had done everything that she could to show Sacha how committed she was to her. They had both gained so much strength from my network of supportive healers, and Alex felt deeply grounded. She could focus now on what was best for Sacha. She knew she had to make a decision, and asked Mia, one of my advanced animal healing students, to conduct one final healing. It was a beautiful experience for both of them, and Mia told me how Sacha became deeply relaxed and settled. She was put to sleep two days later, and is resting in peace in Alex's parents' garden.

Sacha always enjoyed coming to see Liz and couldn't wait to get to the healing centre. We both found the spiritual healing very relaxing and therapeutic. I know Sacha always loved the essential oils, which helped her over the years with all her medical conditions.
ALEX

Behaviour Therapy

If you pick up a starving dog and make him prosperous, he will not bite you. This is the principal difference between a dog and a man.
MARK TWAIN

A lot of my work is to do with behaviour, either the animal's or the owner's. Much of the time, bad behaviour stems from incorrect decision making by the owner. It's often the expectation of the owner that's the issue.

Owners need to be realistic about a pet's needs, and whether or not they are going to be able to fulfil them. Animals are very straightforward, and happily and naturally fall into their packs, herds or groups. Choosing wisely is an essential part of their leadership skills; for example, a collie who chews the furniture while stuck alone in a high-rise flat all day is not a dog with behaviour issues, but a bad choice of breed by the owner. I always say that there is no such thing as a bad animal, just a human who can't lead.

Eileen and Her Greyhounds

Eileen had been having issues with her two rescue greyhounds, Sadie and Arfur. Arfur is the size of a Shetland pony and, although Sadie is more petite, both dogs are extremely powerful. Eileen had been knocked off her feet many times, particularly on walks when trying to restrain them from running off after another dog or animal. Eileen has always loved greyhounds and has rescued them for many years. She is passionate about helping retired greyhounds and cannot imagine living without them. However, since taking retirement she was beginning to doubt her own ability to cope with the situation.

All dogs come with stories, feelings and needs, and it was important to know more about these two before we could look at how Eileen was going to be able to establish a better relationship. As we arranged a time to meet on the phone, Eileen told me that Arfur had been a very successful racing dog in his time but, like many of his breed, once he had outgrown his usefulness, he had been dumped at the local rescue centre. It's a sad reality that where there's a greyhound track, there's usually a greyhound rescue centre. I would love to see a percentage of the dogs' winnings set aside for old racers, but instead they are simply disposed of. I find it disgusting; many of these beautiful dogs have lost their families, their sense of identity and their purpose after years of loyal service.

Sadie was a quiet, inward-looking dog and seemed to mirror Eileen's anxious character. Lack of leadership usually comes from low self-esteem, and Arfur was clearly in charge of this family. Eileen was nervous about bringing the dogs to see me, and confessed that she hadn't even told her husband where she was going. I was clear from the start that this was not on, and nipped her secret visits in the bud. I would need to work with the whole family, I told her; this was a pack issue and anything she took home from the session, such as new commands, would need to be consistently practised by her husband, too. It was important that everyone was playing the same tune.

I understood how Eileen was feeling, but I needed to take a strong lead. She didn't know whom to turn to for help or whether something like healing would even make a difference. I wondered to myself whether leaving work and taking early retirement had knocked Eileen's confidence.

There were clearly other issues going on, and we explored some of the family dynamics in our consultation. Arfur had only been with the family for eight weeks, and although he seemed to be an impressive, confident dog, I could tell that this wasn't the whole story. It didn't take long for Eileen to confess that her husband, Brian, was over-protective of Sadie; she was his girl, and he was a little jealous of Arfur and the enormous presence that he commanded in the household. Arfur clearly adored Sadie and wanted to be her main man.

Eileen was in the middle of all this, feeling at a low ebb as she approached the next stage of her life. She felt disempowered, and that, somehow, the fact that the family dynamics were not gelling was all her fault. It seemed to me that a more normal pack order needed to be established.

It's often said that rescue dogs never forget; I have seen this first hand time and time again in the clinic. Dogs feel deep emotional pain just as strongly as we do, and I really got a sense of how Arfur was feeling when Eileen told me about an incident at the greyhound rescue centre's recent charity event. Eileen had spent hours baking cakes for it and Arfur had sloped off to the cake stall where he had stripped the cakes clean of all the icing. This was unusual behaviour for him and Eileen was not amused. At the show Arfur's reaction was very strange; he was getting more anxious by the minute as other greyhounds were paraded around him, and he growled at any that came near him. When he got home, he refused to eat for days and became very subdued. I could see in our consultation he had lost weight – a clear sign of stress.

I wondered if Arfur had worried that he was going to be given back to the centre, or even to the race track. He did not know this was supposed to be a fun day. Sometimes we need to imagine what it is like from a dog's perspective. Stress sits on the stomach, and I think he became so anxious that he simply could not eat.

I gave Eileen a couple of oils to offer him and we watched as Arfur chose only the rose to sniff rather than to lick, processing the wonderful floral fragrance. I started the healing, and quickly noticed that the heat was mainly in his chest area. His heart felt broken, and he sighed as he absorbed the healing and began to relax right down. Eileen was astonished at how relaxed the dogs were. To her, they had become insurmountable problems, yet here they were now, happily snoozing as I placed my hands next to each of them in turn.

After the healing they were very chilled and so I took the opportunity to offer Eileen a healing, too. She wept quietly as she realized just how stressful her life had become, and I gently encouraged her to let it all go. Sadie looked up to check on her, but she knew that Eileen was in safe hands and, with a sigh, lay down again next to her man.

After the healing we were both feeling very grounded and I suggested that we try taking the dogs for a walk so that I could show her some basic training techniques. Eileen was concerned that they would run after another dog, bowl it over and upset the owner, so I told her that we would go to a field where there were no other dogs and very few distractions. I needed her to change her mindset, so I asked her to join me in a creative visualization as I talked her through exactly what would happen. We imagined the calm serenity of the field where we would be walking with two relaxed, happy dogs walking obediently by our sides. I offered her a vision of the two of us coming back happy, refreshed and feeling that she had achieved something. This is so important: it's so true that energy follows thought. Very often, just thinking positively about an experience can make it happen the way you want it to. Horse riders know that it's important to look beyond an obstacle to encourage a horse to walk on rather than to focus on what's ahead. That will is communicated to the horse as clearly as if the rider had put a pair of blinkers on him.

This would be active training, I told Eileen. She would take Sadie and I would take Arfur on loose leads, keeping their attention on us by changing our pace at certain intervals of the walk, and bringing the focus back if they were distracted by gently touching their rump with a finger, making a 'pshhht' noise each time. There's a real art in correcting something as it happens; there's no point in punishing a dog after the event.

As we walked through the fields behind the clinic, I impressed upon Eileen that the dogs were not doing anything wrong by running off at the sight of a rabbit or a deer, or if they seemed too keen to play with another dog. She needed to understand that their instincts were natural. It was *her* behaviour that needed to change, not theirs. They would obey a pack leader who gave them plenty of opportunity to run, who understood and respected their needs.

Greyhounds have been hunting as sight hounds in the British countryside for more than 400 years, and were bred to lead the Irish wolfhounds and bloodhounds in deer or wild-boar hunts. They are athletes. They see and they chase. Horses are the only other animals that can keep up with greyhounds at 45 mph. Henry VIII loved to take his hounds hunting, with the greyhounds spotting the kill and the hunting dogs such as the labradors, mastiffs and spaniels forming the quarry around the prey. Breeds all had a place in hunting society, and it's no wonder that some have behaviour issues as they settle into the cities and enclosed spaces we've introduced them to in the last century or so.

It's important to understand that, even if we don't hunt with our dogs any more, the instinct is still alive in them. We need to know that the point of the hunt was for man and animal to work together.

I told Eileen how important it is to 'think dog', to know what he would do in the wild and be ready to touch his flank to tell him not to if it is not appropriate. Arfur's ear was ready and cocked, ready for my next command throughout our walk. He was totally connected with me, listening to what I wanted him to do. Sadie was looking happily up at Eileen. It was clear to them who was in charge This natural relationship between human and dog has lasted thousands of years and is something to be honoured rather than feared.

As we chatted, I asked her to look at her own body language. We had been discussing leaders of the pack like Henry VIII and his hunting lords, and Eileen giggled as I pointed out how she was standing, how much lower down in her pack she seemed to be. I told her to stand tall and to be proud of herself, to assume the feeling of pack leader. 'Put your boobs out, Eileen,' I told her, and she burst out laughing and stuck her chest out, tucking her tail bone in and standing with weight equally distributed throughout both sides of the body. I talked her through how to feel her feet rooting into the ground, and she naturally put her shoulders back and looked up and ahead. I took her chin in my hands and told her to relax her arms down, and then gave her some breathing techniques to ground herself whenever she felt her nerves getting the better of her. I felt like Barbara Woodhouse, barking all these orders at her. I told her I bet her that she wouldn't find her vet doing this, and she giggled like a small child all the way back to the clinic.

It was a great start. I was really proud of Eileen and how quickly she had picked up the information. Despite the giggling, we had been completely focused on the dogs, as they were on us. But I'm sure I speak on behalf of a lot of therapists when I say that visualization is not a quick fix, and it's vital that I get a commitment from the pet owner to go the distance. 'Discipline' is a word I often use in the clinic, but this is more about creating healthy boundaries than imposing rules. It's about creating structure. A lot of people shut their dogs away to avoid behaviour issues rather than look at what's happening to make an animal behave in a way that doesn't sit well within the pack. I always tell my clients that this is moral rather than obedience training.

The first thing for Eileen to do now was to find a safe place to take her dogs for a walk, somewhere they would have room to run. She needed more than a back garden for dogs that have been bred to race, but she also needed to be able to get them back when they were off the lead. A good lead would help to keep control, and I suggested a full harness. For this situation I didn't want her to use a halter that covered the nose; a harness that covered the trunk was more appropriate here.

When Eileen and the dogs came back for their second healing session, I wanted to show her how safe it would be for Arfur and Sadie to meet other dogs. Lily, Alf and Morris are used to all kinds of dogs coming into the garden, and I always think of them as part of my healing team. A squat Jack Russell and two little Norfolk terriers would surely prove to Eileen that her dogs were safe with even the smallest of dogs.

We took them into the garden first without leads, and opened the kitchen door for my dogs to run out. Morris meets and greets everyone with such affection, and Arfur and Sadie ran around the garden happily with them right from the start. Greyhounds are such noble dogs and it's lovely to see how gentle big dogs can be with smaller ones.

Eileen had taken everything on board from the last consultation, and we took them all out for a walk this time. Eileen was in charge of Sadie and Alf and I took charge of Arfur, Morris and Lily. Eileen had noted me saying that energy follows thought, and she kept her intentions positive, reaffirming to herself, 'I am a confident pack leader and I am enjoying this walk.' And it was a wonderful walk, with her charges obedient and happy and Eileen feeling deeply empowered by the experience.

As they played with each other, I commented to Eileen that she seemed to be growing with every session. She told me how much more confident she felt, how much more in control of her life she was. She looked at the dogs in a new light these days, respecting their heritage and loving their individual characters. She deeply respected the way that Arfur had bravely managed the enormous sense of loss in his life and was totally committed to ensuring that he and Sadie had what they needed.

Eileen even told her husband about the healing. He had been sceptical at first but when the behaviour of the three other members of his household was transformed so quickly, he was left in no doubt. I invited her to bring him to the follow-up healing sessions, and she was so relieved to find that he loved the healing atmosphere.

These days, both Eileen and her husband come to my healing meditation evenings, and he loves meeting the students who have worked with Sadie and Arfur. He tells them how much of a difference their work has made to all of them, which is wonderful feedback for budding healers to hear.

> It's almost magic the way animals respond to Liz's touch.
> My dogs went from nervous, high-strung creatures,
> traumatized by their pasts, to confident, laid-back and
> fun-loving creatures after one healing session with Liz.
>
> EILEEN

Michele and Gorgeous George

Eileen did what any responsible animal owner would do: she dealt with the difficulties of her situation and found her way through. Her reward was her own self-development – but that wasn't her motivation, and that's so important.

Most cat and dog owners do take full responsibility for their pets. Luckily, in this country it's still not the norm to give a dog to a rescue centre just because he doesn't fit immediately into a lifestyle, but sadly the same cannot be said for some horse owners. Working with animals is like having a child; they need just as much commitment. People don't give their children away if they're hard work, yet the responsibility of keeping a much larger animal, from the cost of feed, stabling, vet and farrier to the workload of turning out and exercise, can lead otherwise responsible people to give up on a horse.

A horse will usually have a number of owners in his lifetime; it's quite normal for a pony to be sold on after his teenage rider has grown out of him, or simply been distracted by life in secondary school after being devoted as a smaller child. It makes me terribly sad when I see the effect of this on some of the horses I treat; they are often so beaten down by life, the result of not being treated with due respect. It's a real challenge to go deeply into some of the psychological issues that many of my horse patients suffer from as they are passed from pillar to post for so much of their lives. Many have had so many demands made upon them with very little given back.

Horses have done so much for us in the course of history, yet we still don't honour them properly. Over eight million horses died in service on all sides in the First World War alone, and in the Second World War we very nearly lost our best European bloodlines. If it wasn't for the heroic people who smuggled a few stallions out from the continent to breed them again before they were left to starve, we wouldn't have some of the extraordinary warmblood breeds we have now.

Horses have always had a job to do while living alongside humans and they have done it willingly. I'm in awe of the way that a horse will tune in to his rider. The horse is one of the few animals on the planet that we actually sit on and become one with. It blows me away that a flight animal can have that amount of trust in a human being, and whether he is show jumping or hacking, that he would so willingly engage with what humans want to do.

I met George, a fabulous Belgian warmblood, back in 2001. At 14 years of age, he was at the peak of his career as a top dressage horse, the beautiful sport of ballet on horseback, with competitions held at all levels from amateur to the Olympics. He had reached the advanced level of Prix St George under the show name of Gorgeous George, in honour of his stunning looks. He was 16.2 hands, chestnut with four white socks and a beautiful white blaze. He was so handsome that the audience would melt as soon as he entered the arena.

After competing for so many years, the stress of top competitions and travelling to shows had worn him down. Mentally, physically, emotionally, he was exhausted. Chloe, his owner, would try to ride him into the dressage arena, but she could tell his heart was not in it any more.

Chloe was very understanding and didn't push it. He had been faithful to her and had served her well from a novice, and she knew that it was time to move on. We all find ourselves in changing circumstances, but it's our responsibility to find a good home if we really do have to let a horse move on. Chloe decided to sell him, but, unlike many of her fellow competitors, she didn't sell him as a dressage horse but as a retired horse suitable only for hacking out on rides through the countryside. She wanted to find him another job, perhaps as a companion to another horse, so when she met Michele, a weekend rider with her own yard who was committed to looking after horses, she knew that she had found George's new home.

Michele had phoned to ask me if I would go down and meet George, to help her decide if he was the right horse for her lovely old boy, Storm, an ex-Queen's Regiment horse who had ridden with the hunt until ringbone had forced his retirement. Now, at 20 years old, he was living out the rest of his life in Michele's fields.

I was overawed by the presence of this enormous horse, George. He was magnificent, a real athlete with that certain quirky something that makes these top achievers so special. But as I looked into his eyes I realized why people call them 'windows to the soul'. George may have had the engine of a Formula One car, but his eyes were pits of despair.

Many top competition horses are stabled for long periods of time when they are not travelling to events, simply because they are worth so much money, and Michele longed to give him the freedom of grazing in a large field and making friends with Storm.

She bonded with him straight away. When Chloe visited Michele's yard to check out George's potential new home, she could see from the way that Michele was talking about her own yard and her own horses that she had found her woman.

Before Michele made her final decision, though, she wanted to have a vet look over him and again asked me to ride him in my sand school while the vet checked for any lameness in walk and his respiratory and heart rates in trot and canter. As I sat on top of him and began to walk him around the school, his sheer power took my breath away. George was really something else. All those years of show jumping with Wow had been like driving a Rolls Royce. Wow was solid, strong and utterly reliable, with enormous presence, but riding George with his thrillingly powerful but ultimately unpredictable horsepower was more like driving a Ferrari.

The vet called out to me to bring him into trot, but as I squeezed him on he suddenly struck up a dressage routine, *passaging* around the school, pointing his front legs out ahead and striking out with his back legs almost in slow motion, before breaking into extended trot down the long side of my school, extending his front legs in long balletic strides and engaging from behind in a striking-out pose! All I could see was two front white socks almost the height of his chin as I gently brought him back to walk. I tried again to get him to trot normally, but this time he puffed himself up and started doing *piaffe*, another dressage move in which he rhythmically marched on the spot. He wasn't playing up; this was an arena and this was what he had always known to do! He was like a robot responding to someone pressing a button. There was no sense of him in it at all.

At that time, I knew very little about dressage and tried desperately to think of the tiny movements in the sitting bones and subtle leg aids that are the signals to a dressage horse, but I quickly gave up and thought about what I would do with my own horses. He had never been put through any show-jumping paces before, so the normal leg and seat aids simply were not working. I decided to put the power of thought to work instead. I let him know that I intended us to go into canter. Relaxed again now that I wasn't thinking of dressage moves, he powered into a beautiful, graceful canter.

We were flying around the school, both of us loving the feeling of letting him go for the first time. He seemed to realize that he could be himself. I wasn't containing him and I had allowed him to open up, to stretch his neck down and relax. I could tell that he was uneven, that he had a slight lameness in his front left foreleg on both reins as I took him in both directions around the school, and Michele and I knew that the vet would not pass him, but she didn't mind. He was going to be happy with her and she would look after him for the rest of his days.

Most people find it hard to get used to retirement, and it was the same for George. He couldn't believe that he was able to go out into the field all day after years of being in a stable, and would stand and stare at the space around him rather than munching on the grass.

He immediately took to Storm. Until now he had only seen other horses from a distance, but now he could be with Storm all day and night, and they nuzzled and groomed each other as if they had been together for ever. He was slowly unwinding, although occasionally he would still perform a perfect *piaffe-passage* on the lane, or jump dramatically if a paper bag blew into the air. Michele would tell me tales about his quirky behaviour every time I went to heal him.

He loved those sessions and soaked up the healing. He was fantastically good-looking before, but his eyes shone brightly now. Despite being 16.2 hands, he had felt small inside, but he knew he was not going back to his old life and the trust was growing. Michele and I realized that he had been putting on a front all this time. It breaks my heart to think about how much pressure he had been under.

I am constantly reminded that horses – and dogs, cats and other animals – never totally forget, and six years later a stressful situation triggered that old habit of inappropriately performing top-level dressage movements. It was Good Friday 2007 and an extraordinarily hot afternoon. I was out in the herb garden, cultivating my herbs in a skimpy bikini top and a pair of shorts and enjoying the warm sunshine when Michele phoned me to tell me that Storm had fallen badly in a ditch on a bridle path nearby while out on a ride with George. She asked me to come down and ride George back home while she and her friend worked with the fire brigade to get Storm out.

I grabbed a riding hat and some chaps and headed off down the lane where I knew they were. As I got there, two fire engines were arriving, their orange lights blazing and sirens wailing. I grabbed hold of George and swung into the saddle and prepared to take him home. But at the sound of two more fire engines arriving and a crane being cranked up, George launched into his stress-induced perfect dressage routine. I concentrated on trying to soothe him, sending him wave after wave of calm thoughts. I blanked out the sounds and sights around me so I could focus on the rhythm of his body movements and becoming one with him. I decided to ride through it rather than against it and concentrated on enjoying the experience rather than mirroring the panicked atmosphere. He was magnificently *piaffing* now, rising up to 18 hands with his high-legged prancing, much to the hilarity of the firemen. I suppose the sight of a bikini-clad woman on top of a dancing horse must have looked pretty funny in the middle of this drama, and I had to fight hard to stay centred while trying to keep George focused as we danced all the way home.

Thankfully Storm recovered from his ordeal, and I am truly grateful to those remarkable firefighters who saved his life. Perhaps the sounds and lights had reminded George of the competition arena and the stress had taken him right back to that robotic behaviour. Unless these psychological issues are brought to the surface, they will be repeated under certain conditions. It's the same for us when we hear an old song that can take us right back to the deep emotions associated with it.

When Liz gives my fabulous retired dressage horse a 'hands-on healing' session, he goes off into a deep, relaxed world, almost nodding off at times, and becomes really chilled out. George self-selects herbal remedies/oils and is just potty with carrot seed oil and peppermint oil, too.

Now, whenever my horses have experienced a somewhat traumatic time, maybe whilst being out on a hack, or if they have injured

themselves slightly while they play in their fields, I call upon Liz for
some help. I know she can assist in their rehabilitation process by
transferring her healing powers and energy into my equines.

MICHELE

Hannah and Rama

If a man aspires toward a righteous life,
his first act of abstinence is from injury to animals.

LEO TOLSTOY

I believe that all animals respond to love, and that any bad behaviour can be corrected, but Rama, the six-year-old Rottweiler, was one of my biggest challenges.

Hannah had rescued him from the kennels where she worked after his previous owners had split up and put him there for re-homing. Although his history was not clear, Hannah suspected that he had been trained to attack, perhaps as a security dog, and he was extremely aggressive to anyone who came towards him, looking directly into their eyes as if he would attack at any moment.

But Hannah had fallen in love with him over the weeks she spent with him; as she pottered around in his cage, chatting away to him as she cleared it out, he would nuzzle her gently. She despaired of him as she watched him turn back into the stereotypical Rottie every time prospective owners approached his cage. It was as if he was willing them to hate him. So Hannah decided to bite the bullet and adopt him herself. How difficult could it be to train a beautiful dog like him?

Hannah had badly misjudged how hard it can be to take on an animal with behaviour issues, and life became very tricky. Rama continued to stare out anyone coming towards him, and hated men in particular. Soon, she was taking him for walks at 5 a.m. to avoid meeting anyone. His moods could switch so quickly, and she lived in fear of him going for someone's throat.

Hannah's whole life revolved around Rama. Even her new boyfriend Paul knew that he had to play second fiddle, and had reservations about Rama's rehabilitation. Her friends couldn't understand her devotion to this apparently psychotic dog who would fix his steely glare on them. She would get dirty looks from other dog owners if she did take him out in public, and she was frequently told that she should have her 'dangerous' dog put down.

Hannah found my number on the internet and rang to ask if I could help. I never turn anyone away, but I admit I did feel a little worried. I had never had a patient like this before and knew I was walking into unknown territory. I trusted that love and lack of judgement would work their magic, but I recognized the need to take real precautions. I asked Hannah to put a metal crate in the boot of the car through which I could make my first contact.

I went out to greet them in the car park. Rama stood like a sumo wrestler, feet square in his crate, locking on to my gaze like the fighter that he was bred to be. But I had prepared myself and I calmly concentrated on sending wave after wave of love towards him. I sat on a chair near the open boot as Hannah and I talked through the consultation form.

Rama was already right at the front of the cage, so I looked away and concentrated on Hannah. I was not being submissive, but I was refusing to give his intimidating stare any energy. I willed myself to stay calm.

Animals pick up on energy and smell the pheromones created by fear. My own flight-or-fight mechanism was alerted; self-preservation kicks in when we're faced with danger and adrenaline was pumping into my system to enable me to flee if necessary. I had to really will myself to override this with positive thoughts. Rama was baring his teeth now and barking aggressively but the crate made me feel more secure, and I focused on getting the oils out of the box and keeping calm.

I chose the rose and handed it to Hannah to offer Rama. So often the first sniff of rose oil will touch a nerve in a distressed animal and send them reeling, and Rama sniffed the bottle and inhaled deeply. He stared into space, his eyes becoming softer by the second and then slumped back, letting out a sigh and resting his huge head on the blanket in the crate.

I let him sniff the violet leaf, then yarrow and then the calendula, which he grabbed with his mouth. I carefully took the bottle back and put a little of the oil on Hannah's finger and he licked and licked. I could tell that he was in heaven. I went on to start the healing from my chair at the entrance to the boot, still without making full eye contact with him. It was very early spring and still very cold, so I wrapped myself up in my coat and tried to ignore the fact that my hands were freezing. I could feel so much pent-up emotional energy in this beautiful dog as he lay there in his crate, sighing gently before going to sleep. Hannah and Paul simply could not believe their eyes.

They brought Rama back to see me every couple of weeks from then on and we went through the same routine with the crate in the back of the car. Hannah was convinced that he associated that crate with a trip to the clinic and would leap into it each time, panting happily. There was no more baring of teeth or aggressive stance. This was a dog who was feeling safe with someone other than Hannah. We had established a positive bond.

On the fourth visit I introduced Rama to my students so that they could practise working from a distance. Safety always comes first, and we all sat around the car with Rama still in his cage and breathed in the enormous gratitude coming from him. By the sixth visit we decided to bring him out of the crate, my students kneeling on the grass on one side of my garden gate and me on a small wooden stool next to it. Hannah was holding Rama on a lead on the other side of the gate. We attuned and began healing.

Rama calmly backed his bottom into my hands through the gate and I felt his warm fur for the first time, and affectionately scratched his back through the wooden slats. He didn't flinch, but lay down as close as he could get to the gate. The healing energy and positive intentions from all of us were creating an even bigger trust now and with every subsequent visit, his progress was astonishing. He really wanted to be a happy, loving dog. It felt to us that he had been misunderstood for so much of his life.

Rama came to me for about a year and became more and more relaxed over that time. And as he calmed down, Hannah became more assertive; she expected Rama to follow her commands now rather than simply hoping in vain. Paul had been her rock, showing tremendous support and dedication to this lengthy training. There is so much love and devotion between Hannah, Paul and Rama that I feel confident that Rama will continue to grow into the dog that Hannah somehow always knew he was. Because Hannah had absolute belief in his rehabilitation, she had helped Rama to heal himself.

> *Elizabeth can look beyond the troubled exterior of a dog-and-human partnership and see what truly lies within – without doling out textbook behavioural advice. Thank you, Liz, for your compassion.*
> HANNAH

All You Need Is Love

At the risk of sounding like a song lyric, I've found over the last decade of healing animals that love is all they really need from their owners. This is where my healing philosophy starts and finishes. What so many of my clients and pet patients discover through their journey of healing is an astonishing commitment to each other, something that they will cherish and remember for the rest of their lives.

We could learn a thing or two from our pets: animals have a capacity for unconditional love that is breathtaking, and I feel really privileged to see it every day in my clinic. Regardless of species or issues that come to my couch, the story is always the same: an animal never expects anything in return but is happy to give in bucketfuls. Imagine what we could be if we could love like them.

I try to teach all my clients that this kind of unconditional love really can make a great difference to their pet. Even the sickest animal will brighten up if his owner can make the shift from fear and anxiety to love and acceptance. I've noticed time and time again how energy follows thought, how thinking differently, positively, really can improve any situation, however hopeless it may seem.

Brenda and Teddie

Teddie was a German Spitz dog, part of the toy family and one of seven Spitze in Brenda's home. He was born with an open fontanelle (the soft area on the top of the head) where his bone tissue had not completely formed.

This would normally mean that a dog would be prone to brain damage and have a very low life expectancy, and when Teddie came to me at five months old he had already begun to lose his coordination and to sleep most of the day. He was very tiny and had so little interest in food that Brenda had to feed him by hand. Brenda's vet had suggested steroids for the inflammation on the brain, but warned that it would be highly unlikely that Teddie would ever come off the medication. The slightest knock could also cause further brain disease.

Brenda knew the full implications of long-term steroid use and decided not to pursue this course of action, but she refused to give up on Teddie and – just as importantly – to let him know that she was worried. Instead, she went to a holistic vet who supported Teddie's needs with homeopathic treatments for a while. Intuitively, though, Brenda felt that something was missing from the treatment. She already believed in the benefits of animal healing, so when her daughter-in-law picked up my details at an animal healing talk, she gave me a call.

When she first brought him to me, Teddie was like a little ginger rag doll in her arms, his big eyes looking out at me from his limp, fluffy body. After a full consultation, we put him on the carpet to see just how much he could move, but he just lay there, looking up at us in resignation. Brenda scooped him back into her arms as I offered him some oils. I took out the bottle of violet leaf, a rich green liquid with a leafy aroma, and he sniffed it carefully and took a couple of licks of it from her finger.

Violet leaf is a grounding oil for fear of new places and uncertainty, and is very often an oil which animals will choose when they first come to me for a healing.

Not all essential oils are made from the flower heads, as you might think; some are made from roots, others from leaves, and others from resins. If you think of a violet, you might think of the beautiful velvety flower which you find close to the ground. But if you look at how big the leaf is compared to the flower, you'll see that it acts as its protector. Zoopharmacognosy refers to this as 'the doctrine of signatures', the visual interpretation of a name. This is one of the ways in which humans differ from animals: we tend to overlook medicinal plants which we might not have seen before, while animals make their choices largely by smell. In the wild, animals would easily find their way to this natural medicine cupboard. I believe that as we have taken them into captivity, it's our responsibility as their caretakers to understand just how Nature can still meet their needs. It's all about giving something back to them and being humble enough to recognize that their instincts haven't been depleted in the way that ours have.

Teddie continued to sniff the oils, and was very interested in the yarrow, so I poured a little on Brenda's finger and he licked it gently. When taken internally, the flavonoid constituents of yarrow act to strengthen blood vessels at the extremities and help remove small blood clots. He then chose the carrot seed, which is great for cell damage and is an immune-stimulant. The essential oil is distilled from the fruits of wild carrot rather than the tuber so there's no point in trying this with something from your vegetable box. Self-selection is not something that anyone should try at home; even dabbling with tea tree oil on its own, for example, can burn the skin.

I was astonished as Teddie used both sides of his tongue to lick up the carrot seed. I checked in my Caroline Ingraham book and he was right: the sub-lingual (under-the-tongue) absorption of oils is more effective for getting them into the bloodstream. I knew that homeopathic pills are popped under the tongue for this reason, but I couldn't believe that Teddie would know to do this. Working with animals is a constant reminder of how much more they know than us about Nature's products.

I noted down that Teddie loved the seaweed oil. In its form of kelp it is known to help humans with arthritis, nerve and muscle function, and its zinc supports the nervous system. This was just what he needed. He deeply inhaled bergamot, an oil for depression and balancing the emotions, and looked deep in thought before turning his head away, so I offered him yellow birch, an anti-inflammatory and analgesic which inhibits blood clotting. Again, he licked some off Brenda's finger and loved it.

I also offered him peppermint, a stimulant which I only ever offer at the end of a session because it activates the nerve pathways and is particularly helpful for animals with limited movement; Teddie had muscle atrophy as a result of his paralysis and his limbs were already withering. He was clearly enjoying himself now, licking his lips and focusing completely on what was being offered. This was so different from anything that he had ever had before for his disability.

We settled into the healing and noticed that Teddie's legs were already stretching out a little. He was now on the floor, still in Brenda's arms. I asked her if she would let him try to move by himself. She was reluctant because she didn't want to be disappointed, but Teddie had other ideas. He amazed us all by slowly crawling a metre or so across the floor. I stood him up to relieve the pressure on his organs and gently took my hands away. He stood up for a couple of moments by himself before gently folding down again. It was a real breakthrough.

In the wild, Teddie's condition would be a critical weakness, and left to his own devices he would try to heal himself by using his powerful sense of smell to find his own medicines. Being treated by humans must have been disempowering for him, but this was a team effort now and for Brenda to watch him self-select his own medicine was a reminder of how instinctive her beautiful dog still was. The moment she walked into the room, I had a gut feeling that I would be seeing a lot more of her; the way that she understood what healing was about and her utter devotion to her dogs showed me what a healer she was, too. It's no surprise to me that she is now a graduate of my animal healing course.

We arranged more sessions and I began to bottle up the five remedies that Teddie had chosen. I always offer the animals the opportunity to self-select the base oil before making up the individual remedies, and Teddie had chosen sunflower oil. I added a couple of drops of the essential oils he had selected and gave precise instructions on the order in which they should be offered. Each bottle was clearly labelled, and Brenda agreed that she would follow my instructions.

Brenda was one of the most committed clients I have ever had, and came to see me every two weeks. She knew that the treatment was truly holistic and that the atmosphere at home, the oils and Teddie's diet were just as important as the healing. Brenda is a woman after my own heart when it comes to food, and her dogs were already being fed a home-cooked diet of fresh meat, fish, vegetables and pulses. She completely understood the nutritional value of real food.

Each session, we would go through the same self-selection process. There were times when Teddie would only sniff the aromas or turn his head away. As we only reach for a paracetamol (or chew on a feverfew leaf or two) when we have a headache, so an animal only selects a remedy when he needs it. None of us continues with the pain relief when the headache is gone.

Sometimes I prepare remedies that animals have self-selected in a consultation only to find that the owners have given up offering them because their pet has only sniffed at them. I remind them that inhaling is just as important as licking, and animals know this. They will only ever do what they need to do. But Brenda was not one of those clients, and her observation notes were perfectly detailed. She had made a commitment to follow through the treatments, which is incredibly important.

Within two months, Teddie was not only up on his feet but pottering around the garden on his own. Brenda told me that Teddie was so happy in himself that he often seemed to be smiling at her. Every time she presented the oils for him to self-select, he would go into a frenzy of excitement. I had trained Brenda to give him regular healings, and she reported back that he had regained full use of his legs and was one of the pack again. When he was tired, Brenda would carry him, but Teddie's self-esteem was high and he was clearly enjoying a full and active life.

Despite the short life expectancy of dogs with open fontanelles, Teddie lived a happy life until he passed away just before his third birthday. He had a fantastic relationship with Brenda and the other dogs, and she knew that she could not have done any more to give him such happiness in his short life. I believe that it was her intention to help him heal himself and her commitment to the treatment that were paramount in making his life such a happy one.

Elizabeth is a dedicated, warm and inspirational person who unconditionally gives healing energy to all animals and people alike. She changed my life and Teddie's with her generous, loving spirit. Teddie just blossomed after each healing treatment and oils. He reached his full potential and, above all, was so, so happy. He filled my life with love.
BRENDA

Intention

A dog has the soul of a philosopher.
PLATO

Like all sentient beings, pets will drink up the emotions of others – especially of their owners – and feel an enormous responsibility to heal their owners' grief or loneliness. Recognizing the impact that their own stress and life choices have on their pets is stage one in the recovery process – for both owner and pet. So many people who come through my door with their animal's condition leave with a fundamental shift in their own world view. Over a course of treatment at the clinic, many of my clients find that taking responsibility for their own feelings allows them to take a new view of the way that they live their lives. For some, this can be literally life changing.

Holly and Wow

I met 21-year-old Holly through her lovely dogs Millie and Ruby, a mother-and-daughter pair of whippet cross rescue dogs which Holly and her mum, Gill, brought to my Tuesday night animal healing evening. They had heard about the evening and hoped that learning how to meditate and relax using creative visualization and group healing might help Ruby's lethargy and stiffening joints and Millie's excessive hair loss.

It's interesting how often animals bring an issue to me that reflects their owners', and the parallels didn't escape me here. I had noticed the dynamic between human mother and daughter, and wondered what it was that was making Gill so exhausted.

I was pleased when she took me aside after the group and asked me if she could book a treatment for the dogs, and a few days later we met again for a full consultation. I suggested that the dogs' diet of mainly dry food was the first thing to change and I offered oils and conducted a healing. As the atmosphere in the room became still and the dogs relaxed right down, I noticed that Gill was finding it hard to hold back the tears. I passed her some tissues and encouraged her to let the burden off her shoulders, but quickly realized that with Holly in the room, this was not the time.

Later, as Holly was playing with the dogs in the garden, Gill told me how impressed she had been with the healing on the dogs and sheepishly asked if I could offer something similar to Holly. I laughed and told her that I was trained as a human healer too and it wasn't such an odd suggestion, that lots of the animals' owners come to me for healing. In fact, I suggested, she should come too!

By the time Gill came to me for her own healing, her dogs were as right as rain and I could tell that she was hoping to achieve this herself. She told me that Holly had had epilepsy since she was a baby of six months. She and her twin sister had had the triple vaccination (MMR: measles/mumps/rubella) at the same time and while Amy was fine, Holly had become ill almost immediately. No one will ever know if a link can be proven, but Holly contracted a cortical brain problem which reduced her sight to tunnel vision. Over a period of time her sight recovered a little and by age nine she was able to have an operation to correct the remaining squint. This successful eye operation proved the wonders of conventional medicine for her and restored her sight completely. Her coordination problems were less easy to fix, though. Her parents, who were totally committed to getting the best care for her that they could afford, had spent years doing everything to address this.

Holly and Gill both came to me for regular healings, and over the next few months I learned a little more about their lives. Holly had been through state primary school, with the inevitable bullying that little children who appear to be different will suffer, and a special school where she had been almost mute despite regular speech therapy. Her epilepsy had been managed by regular diagnostic treatment with EEGs and the brilliant drug, Epilim, but she was still completely out of control of her own body and had no idea when she might experience another episode. Living an ordinary life was almost impossible. When I met her she had been stacking shelves in a local supermarket for work experience, and although she was supervised she had been told after two weeks that she was 'not right for the job'.

Holly and I had discovered an instant rapport and I looked forward to her sessions enormously. She is a very beautiful girl but terribly shy, and I felt for her when she told me that her twin is a stunner and very outgoing. I wondered what I could do for Holly other than the healing. I noticed that she had taken to Wow in a big way, often chatting to him for an hour or more over the stable door while Gill was having her treatment. I gently suggested that she come and spend some more time with him.

I knew that Wow could heal Holly, while giving Gill the break that she so badly needed. Animals are so much less complicated than we are, so much more present. They don't make judgements about disability or worry about 'what if…?' Their warmth and pure love seem to make the world a better place for a while. Scientists have even proven that stroking cats can reduce stress levels. Apparently in Tokyo, one company even encourages workers to stroke cats during their breaks to increase staff morale and productivity. Animals are natural healers; look at the way pets bring out the smiles and raise the spirits when allowed into old people's homes, how very often it's their uncomplicated and unconditional love that makes them more welcome visitors than the friends and family who have brought them in.

Right from the first, Holly seemed to develop a love affair with horses. She adored all of mine, but Wow, despite being a massive 16.3 hands, was her favourite. He was a gentleman with her and dropped his normal habit of having a little nibble and a sniff when he's with new people, nuzzling her gently instead. She told me recently, 'He seems to know that he needs to look after me. He's my best friend.'

I encouraged her to groom him in the stable itself, knowing that they would get so much pleasure from each other without the stable door between them. Being with such a big horse in such a small space could well have been daunting, but Wow would nuzzle Holly's hair gently as she was brushing him and seemed to me to glow with pride and love when he was with her. She had never experienced anything like this before and was clearly enjoying this one-to-one relationship.

After a few weeks of observing them together, I asked Holly if she would like to try sitting on him. Her initial reluctance and deep-seated fear were totally understandable and I let the thought sink in for a couple of days before trying again. She was petrified that she would have a seizure while in the saddle. This was a girl who had worn a crash helmet throughout her life in case she had a seizure and the thought of falling from such a height was terrifying.

I had already taught her a lot about breath work in her healing sessions, and I reminded her of how she could use this to get over her fear. Finally, she agreed. Wow stood as still as a rock with Gill and me standing at his side, and with the help of a large mounting block, Holly struggled into the saddle. I coached her through the breathing, holding Wow with a secure lead rein attached to the bridle as Wow and Holly made their first journey together around my sand school.

She had a beautiful position and sat naturally in the saddle. She was generous and light with her reins with a good leg position so that Wow could easily feel her as she squeezed into his flank to indicate a turn. She was a naturally sympathetic horse rider, going with his rhythm rather than imposing hers on him. She had learned how to ride some time ago but was reluctant to continue in case her condition held her back. She was even worried that some people might find her too slow. I watched in astonishment as this timid, fearful young woman seemed to rise in stature on my beautiful horse.

After six sessions in the sand school, she had become confident enough to go out on a brief hack up the lane with Dancer, Gill, Ruby and Millie and me all by her side. The dogs were clearly thrilled to see their young mistress so happy, and I realized that part of their original depression may have been around Holly's lack of enthusiasm for life. Like many teens, she had never really been interested in taking them for a walk, but the toll her own depression was taking on the rest of the family had spread to the dogs. As they trotted along behind her now, their tails wagging, I realized that this new, exciting hobby of hers could involve the whole family.

She was exhausted when we got back but totally exhilarated, and her smile said it all. I promised her plenty more opportunities to ride and, in return, she offered to do a bit of poo-picking and other odd jobs around the tack room. She couldn't get enough of Wow, and wanted to do as much as she could for him.

Gill was also having a new lease of life; since Holly had left school she had become a full-time carer, and this new routine was giving her a chance to leave Holly with me and have a life of her own for a couple of hours every week.

Although Holly was doing so well, this was no miracle cure, and none of us was surprised when she slipped off the mounting block one day and had a seizure. Her father Peter was with her and was quick to call the paramedics, who were wonderful and set up a mini-hospital at the sand school. Unsurprisingly, although she was fine, Holly's confidence was badly dented.

I needed to get her back on Wow as soon as possible and carefully worked with her, using visualization to prepare her. However terrified she was, she trusted me and Wow enough and, after a few days, she was in the saddle again.

I was with her when she thought she was going to have a seizure and was able to see clearly the relationship between her epilepsy and her mindset. She was getting onto Wow one afternoon, who was usually as still as a statue, but on this day he took one step forward. Holly panicked and began to hyperventilate, screaming at me that she was about to have a seizure. I told her to focus on me, to breathe deeply, to tell herself that she would be fine as she climbed down.

As she calmed down and realized that the worst hadn't happened, that she hadn't had a seizure, that she had kept in control, I saw what this was about. She believed that if she fell, she would go into a seizure; it was what she had believed all her life. The crash helmet that I had her seen her wearing in photos from her toddler to teenage years was a physical reminder that if she knocked her head, she would have a seizure. I had to change that way of thinking.

Luckily, my assistant Amanda turned up at that moment and I quickly asked her to hold Wow while Holly got on. I had to get her up there now if she was ever to ride again. Holly blanched, but I talked her through what would happen, bit by bit, how Amanda was going to hold Wow, how she would get onto the mounting block and put her left foot in the stirrup, talking her through every movement until she was in the saddle. Every moment that she would get fearful, I would bring her back to the present, breathing, seeing the outcome as being successful. Wow stood stock-still. He wasn't reacting to her fear. He wasn't mirroring her; he was mirroring me and my composure.

By the time Holly was in the saddle she was smiling, tears of joy pouring down her cheeks, and she let me lead her around the sand school for a full 15 minutes. She kept telling me that this was the most important thing that had ever happened to her. She had achieved something that she had never believed possible.

Holly rode Wow over the next weeks and months with a new confidence. I was thrilled, and wanted to push her even further to take some more responsibility. I felt intuitively that she really needed to find her voice. (She had never talked very much and, when she did, her speech was faltering and weak.)

Then I had an idea. I had recently got into dressage with my younger horse, Dancer, and I needed someone to read the dressage sheets out to me as I practised the moves. The sheets give the instructions for the competition, so it is important they are read loudly, clearly and in time, so I asked Holly if she would like to do this for me. She was very reticent at first, her little voice barely audible over the wind and the clump of hooves on the sand in the school, but I kept encouraging her to shout at me, and over the next few months, with some coaching in voice projection from me, she seemed to grow again as her voice became clearer and stronger.

These days Holly comes with me to dressage competitions and we work as a team. This is a girl who could barely say hello last year and now she stands in front of an audience and a judge reading the test sheets, having coordinated where I am in the routine and anticipated my next move. I don't compete very often due to my work commitments, but when I have an opportunity to do something for me, I relish the chance to be with my horses and Holly. It is challenging, and when we perform at a dressage competition I admit that it can be nerve-racking for me. Serious competitors and horses are the equivalent of human athletes, and that can be very daunting – but Holly settles my nerves with the new authority in her voice. Of course, she does sometimes get it wrong, but I don't do the competitions for anything other than fun these days and we get through it. It is really important to me that Dancer is enjoying himself, too. He loves meeting other horses and the variety of it all. It's like going to a party for him! Holly is immensely pleased to be able to be part of this.

Holly is so proud of herself, and I am so proud of her. She even came with me to a Health and Healing Festival recently in Buxton, Derbyshire. Iris, our little foal, had just been born and I needed help organizing my lectures and selling CDs and so I asked Holly if she would take responsibility for my till. This was the first time she had been away on her own for any length of time. It's hard work for anyone to spend six hours in the car, but she coped really well and we had a fabulous girls' weekend away. She came to my animal healing workshop and looked after Jake, a beautiful border terrier who was part of the programme, and she loved it. And at the wrap party for all the exhibitors at the end of the show, she even got up and danced with the Urban Gypsies, the belly dancers from *Britain's Got Talent!* She loved it.

Holly is now part of my team at the stables. She was my assistant on the shoot for the photos in this book and helped me bathe Wow at 6 a.m. for the shoot. She was so excited that he was being recognized in this way. She hasn't had a fit now for 12 months and describes herself as feeling self-assured and confident.

My dogs Millie and Ruby are both now old ladies, and Ruby particularly suffers from arthritic joints. Both dogs, even Millie, the more nervous and anxious of the two, visibly relax and settle under Liz's healing touch. This wonderful energy has the same effect on my daughter: as Holly herself says, 'Liz's healing makes me feel so relaxed, I usually fall asleep. Afterwards my head feels clear and I feel stronger in my body.'

GILL

PART THREE
The Travelling Clinic

We can judge the heart of man by his treatment of animals.
IMMANUEL KANT

Mary and Sammy

I see many pets outside the clinic on home visits, and it's lovely to be able to be out and about to see my clients in their own environment. It's so important to be able to see how they live and to show owners how easy it is to heal their own pets themselves. Kneeling on the floor in their own sitting room can be all the inspiration they need to want to try it out for themselves. It's a privilege to be able to see into so many people's lives, to gain a deeper understanding of the human condition, with all its incredible twists and turns.

Some of my clients feel very alone, yet their dog, cat, horse or guinea pig is the one friend in their lives who knows exactly what's going on and what to do about it. Very often we have a best friend under our nose that we haven't even noticed.

Sammy is a beautiful male ginger guinea pig living with a harem of 11 girl guineas in a bungalow near the seaside. His owner, Mary, had called me in to see him because the vet had diagnosed lymphoma, the malignant proliferation of lymphoid tissue under the armpit area. Mary was beside herself; her guineas were her life, and she was devastated to think that she could lose him.

I arrived at Mary's house and knocked on the door. I could see someone at the end of the corridor, hesitating to answer. Finally a shy little sparrow of a woman opened the door and timidly invited me in, apologizing all the time for the mess and for taking up my time. Until recently she had been living there with her invalid mother, who had died six months previously. I sensed that Mary felt awkward about me coming into her home and that she preferred her reclusive life where she could grieve in peace.

The house was immaculate, and I couldn't work out where in this small bungalow the guineas could be kept. She showed me into a double bedroom at the end of the house and, as we opened the door, a chorus of squeaks welcomed us in.

In the wild, guinea pigs, as with all animals, would roam relatively free, and since we have invited their ancestors into our homes, it is important to make sure that we provide the best conditions in the most natural way that we can. Hutches should be big enough for them to move around in, with fresh hay that has not turned mouldy. It is not just a question of providing food and water; good holistic living includes mental stimulation, a good diet to create a strong immune system, exercise, appropriate living conditions and proper companionship.

Mary's guinea home environment was the best example I had ever seen. Their room was light and well ventilated and their food was excellent quality. I sniffed the hay, which was sweet and fresh. It's vitally important that small furries eat fresh hay; if it's old, it gets musty and it can cause respiratory problems. It's also very important that they get a diet rich in vitamin C, and I could see broccoli, tomatoes, spinach, green pepper and cucumber laid out for them. I was also pleased to see that Mary had a good-quality guinea-pig mix, which is also really important. I've had calls from owners of rabbits and guineas to say that their pets' urine is almost fluorescent in colour. Some mixes have so much artificial colouring in them that it comes right through the system. But not so with these guineas. I was really impressed by the way that Mary was looking after them; it was obviously a full-time job.

I also felt I had arrived at the Crufts for small furries! There was every size and colour of guinea pig I had ever seen. There were smooth-coated, short-haired, long-haired, rough-haired, a woolly-haired Rex, and a gorgeous hedgehog-coloured one who was a real babe. Another was white and tan, another a beautifully smooth, glossy-coated furry who looked like something out of a shampoo advert. There was a stunning jet-black baby, another that looked like Dougal from the *Magic Roundabout* (complete with a line all the way down her back) and a smooth otter-coloured one. And there in the middle of all these stunning sows was Sammy. I knew instantly that he was the male. He was tan, with a fabulous punk-rocker hairdo. He was smashing, absolutely gorgeous.

They were all rescue guineas and Mary took great pleasure in telling me about why she had placed one with another. Each had its story; they all came from different places and for different reasons. Very often kids love guineas and other small furries, but as school and friends take priority they lose interest, and parents, who no longer know what to do with the pets, tend to find a rescue home for them.

As we came in, they all stopped munching their hay and greens and looked up at me, their little ears flapping. It was as if they were saying 'Hi!' The guineas were all in different runs, with two or three in each. Sammy was in the central one with two of the most beautiful girls. I could see that they were all extremely happy as they darted in and out of their hay homes. Mary warned me that Sammy would be very difficult to catch, but as I put my hand down to him, he simply walked forward as if he had been waiting to be picked up. All the girls stopped what they were doing, their eyes on me, some standing on their hind legs to see what was happening, and as they settled down I let Sammy make himself comfortable on my lap.

Mary watched amazed as he turned himself round so that his bottom was facing me and looked directly at her for the first ten minutes. As I placed my hands around his body, he soaked up the healing and then, when he felt that he was done on that side, he turned around and nestled his face into my hand so I could tend to his other side.

Mary had cared for guinea pigs for 20 years, and it became clear that they had helped her avoid any other major relationships in her life, other than with her mother. When Sammy had developed a malignant lump under his armpit, it meant an enormous amount to her, and she was keen to ensure that her vet understood the complementary treatment that I was giving him; she was investing everything in these little animals.

From that point, I visited the 'family' every two weeks for healings and advice on diet. A couple of the girls had cystitis and, since the vet's conventional treatment was proving to be a bit hit-and-miss, Mary had asked him if she could try aloe after reading about its cool and soothing effects in a magazine. With the vet's blessing, I made up a gel of fresh aloe vera leaf, including the sap, and mixed a small amount of yarrow in with it before putting a tiny bit on the underside of the sows, being very careful to keep a safe distance from the genitals.

The more time I spent with Mary, the more she opened up. She was still worried that she was taking too much of my time, but I loved the fact that I was making so much of a difference to her life. By now, she was waiting at the door as soon as she heard my car draw up.

She seemed to enjoy the chats over a cup of tea after the healing, and even bought me organic biscuits. She wouldn't spend any money on herself at all; she would eat toast and Marmite while her guineas were eating organic broccoli and I was sipping my Clipper tea, but over the weeks I spent there, with my encouragement, she began to take a look at her own life.

After a while, my visits became less frequent. Mary was eating better and was filling out a little. She was happier and was even making friends with her neighbours. When I last checked up on her, Sammy was not only doing well but Mary was raising money for local rescue centres. This was a woman who never went out except to go to the supermarket.

We all have a voice. We are meant to communicate with each other, but Mary hadn't spoken to anyone for such a long time. She had forgotten how to be in the outside world. It was Sammy who brought that back to her. His illness had been a catalyst in her being able to find a new life after her mother's death.

Animals like to play an important role in our lives. Instead of being a bit-part player, they can feel a real sense of place if given the opportunity. Mostly, they like to ground us, encouraging us to play, to go for walks, to remember what it feels like to run around and have fun. It's unpleasant to feel stressed; our behaviour becomes unreliable, our tempers volatile and our spirit depressed. Our moods swing and, after weeks of heart to hearts, our friends often give us a wide berth until we sort ourselves out. What we need is an anchor in the storm, and our pets are only too happy to offer that to us.

Distant Healing

In the past few years I've begun to pass on some of my healing skills with the aim of spreading my work across the globe. My students are graduating every year now from a one-year diploma in animal healing, and I am stretching my own wings and working with rescue centres and sanctuaries all over the world. But there are also many animals who need care and attention but whom I can't physically get to.

Distant healing can bridge the gap extremely effectively, and with my growing network of healers it is proving a remarkably powerful way of using our collective consciousness to heal animals all over the world. We include wild animals and focus on endangered species in particular.

Very often we are all in different places, yet we experience a wonderful peace among us while we're healing. People talk about group meditations raising vibrations, and we all regularly report feeling a kind of euphoria. You only have to go to a football match or a wedding to see what happens when a large group of people focus their energy on one thing. Even a funeral can allow people to cry and grieve collectively, which can be wonderfully cathartic. It makes you feel good. It seems that distance doesn't break this magic.

But I think it is more than this; I believe that in bringing healing to an individual we are also bringing healing to the universe as a whole, that we and our animals are all inter-connected. The act of healing works like ripples in a pool, reaching out to touch everyone and everything around us. People really like to do things for the highest good, and if they feel that they really are making an impact, not just on an animal's life but on the entire universe, it makes them feel even more connected to each other and to the planet.

There is no mystery in distant healing. As with meditation, it's simply about finding the time in your day to switch the phones off, tell everyone who needs to know that you're not to be disturbed for the next half hour or so, and making yourself comfortable. For me, distant healing is like any other consultation and I'll treat it as such. I book it into my clinic day. I don't charge for it, but it's in my diary for every day.

I use my meditation room and close the door, light the candles and make myself comfortable. Sometimes my three dogs come in, too; they seem to know when I'm healing and come and settle down quietly next to me.

As I start the grounding exercise that always precedes a meditation, I look at my distant healing book in front of me with a list of names of animals and their owners. I can be healing many animals in one session and I don't want to break my concentration by trying to remember the name of the ginger cat from Glasgow that I've forgotten.

I like to work with photographs of the animals and their owners, although some people do find that they can focus better when their eyes are closed. Once I'm grounded and attuned, I take a moment to be really present. I can feel that love bursting from every cell in my body. It feels very special being a channel of love and I give thanks to God.

Any healing is about intention, the focus of one person who is sending positive thoughts to another, and it's vital that the healer feels good and positive so that that energy is projected out into the world. The act of healing itself does us good of course, but during the attunement it's really important that the healer is checking how he or she is feeling and taking responsibility for any feelings before sending out any energy.

Once done, I'm ready to work. I say a little prayer, and begin to visualize the animals and their humans on my list basking in a laser beam of healing light pulsing out of me towards them. I see them well and happy and send the healing to wherever it is needed for them, whether it is physically emotionally, mentally or spiritually. I rhythmically read from my list of names, the pulse of love accompanying each person and animal. I do this out loud, but it's also fine to do this silently.

I make sure that it is love that I'm pulsing rather than sadness or sympathy. I never think about the trauma or the issue, but simply the animal and the family around him. I am often asked to do distant healing on an animal as it is being put to sleep, and sometimes I really have to hold it together. I have to be a very clear channel of energy and often that can take quite some focusing. Some of my patients have been with me for years and I have built up a strong relationship with the owner and pet. I feel their grief but my focus is always on love.

After I've read the names on the list, I extend my love to all the endangered species in the world for a moment. Meditation is all about connecting with the universe and it's important to send that love out to as many beings as I can. For me, healing the animals whose families have asked for it by phone, letter or email is only part of the highest good that I believe distant healing can achieve.

Finally, it's time to come out of the healing and to bring my attention back to the room. I give thanks again to God, to myself and to all the animals I've been working with before drawing all that energy back inside me and regaining full consciousness. Closing down the meditation is part of the routine, just like switching a light off when leaving a room.

If I don't do it, it feels like I'm walking down Oxford Street without any clothes on!

People have their own ways of doing it but I breathe in and visualize all that lovely energy coming back in and around me. I tend to use the lotus flower as a visual aid, closing its petals around a loose bud, protecting the heart of it. I also focus on breathing in a gorgeous gold colour and showering myself with a stardust of gold confetti. It's a euphoric feeling, like a firework going off. It's a wonderful gift to be able to give myself, and this is the moment to really bathe in that feeling. Finally, I gently sink my feet a little deeper into the carpet to ground myself again.

Sitting down and simply focusing on a sick animal, even if he is on the other side of the country, can send enough love to him to begin the healing process. If, as with some of my more committed clients, the intention is hands-on healing at the same time, the combination of distant healing and the client's healing can be truly miraculous.

Sally and Woody

As so many of my students are taking their animal healing diplomas out into the world and doing distant healing themselves, I hear many stories about what can be achieved these days. My favourite, though, is about a dog I healed recently in Northern Ireland. I've still never met him or his owner, but Sally and I have struck up a wonderful phone relationship through my healing work with them both.

Sally called me late one night to tell me about Woody. He had lost a tremendous amount of blood through nosebleeds and she was desperately worried about how weak he was. Her vet had done everything that he could, and had suggested that it would be kinder to put him down. I remember that call: Sally was so low. She couldn't bear the thought of her dog being so weak, but she just couldn't lose him.

There was no way I could get to Northern Ireland regularly enough, so I offered her a one-on-one distant healing by phone at a designated time. We did the consultation form by email, and I could see from his history that Woody had suffered from an immune deficiency. He had been suffering from allergic broncho-pulmonary aspergillosis, which is usually caused by the inhalation of airborne fungal spores that settle and grow in damaged parts of the lung. Blood blisters had then developed in his nose, and these had burst, causing him to lose pints of blood.

People don't think of animals suffering from immune issues, yet one in three children in the Western world is suffering from asthma and eczema, which is usually caused by immune deficiency. I see the same thing in cats and dogs all the time. Small furries don't tend to suffer as much from this because they don't live long enough to develop the disease. You can see just how much it has influenced the animal-food industry: where once shelves in pet shops were lined with tinned dog food, there are now hundreds of different brands featuring everything from gluten-free foods to special diets for hyperactive animals.

Woody's diet was dried, and the most economical brand the supermarket offered. I advised Sally that dogs need a much more varied diet, but that Woody in particular needed foods that would boost his immune system, such as eggs, sardines, chicken, offal and vegetables. She had never thought about giving him the kind of food she gave her family, and reminded me that she was on a very tight budget. I persuaded her to give him some of the food left over from the family dinner and to try cooking a bit extra for a trial period to see how much more expensive it would be. Sally would have done anything for her dog and agreed to try.

As she told me more about herself, I wasn't surprised to hear that she was experiencing difficulties in her own life. She had recently separated from her husband, although he still lived nearby so that he could visit their two children as well as Woody. They both loved the dog, but it is incredibly hard to create a positive atmosphere when you're trying to agree visiting rights; most owners don't recognize the grief felt by the animal itself. Most animals are territorial, and Woody hated spending half the week at one family home and half at another. He was obviously feeling confused about where he needed to be. He felt torn about whom he should be with, and his shortness of breath suggested that he was clearly stressed. Like us, dogs need to have a place they can call home.

I asked her to send me a picture of Woody, with her and her ex-partner's name and phone number on the back. I could tell that she felt better just having something positive to do. She told me that she had always been interested in healing and had always wanted to find someone who could show her how to do it herself. I could see that Sally was taking responsibility for Woody's healthcare now. She wasn't after a quick fix. Many of my clients could read up about their pet's illness or learn about healing themselves, but often they just want someone to talk to and to listen to them. Others say to me, 'I don't care what you do; I just want you to heal him.' Sally was different, and as I took her through a guided meditation on the telephone I gave her a list of things that she could do, too. I gave her a dedicated time when we could do the healing together, and I could tell she was thrilled to get involved. There's a positive energy around taking charge of a situation when you have felt so helpless and vulnerable. You heal yourself and the world follows. People can come into the clinic or talk to me on the phone and it's fine, but when they come to the party, too, the effect can be nuclear.

Although I didn't know this woman, it felt like I was talking to my sister. I'm very at home talking to people on the phone and I love to help others help themselves and change the way they look at the situation. When the owner first comes to me or phones me, he or she is obviously distressed about the illness itself, but I do a gentle healing even as I'm chatting. It's the intention to spread positive thoughts that heals. I always feel that a phone call is about taking the time to give some love, whoever is on the receiving end.

Even though I had a picture of Woody, I still had no idea what Sally looked like. After our first distant healing session on the phone, she told me that she had felt the empathy flooding from me. She was amazed to find Woody coming into the room as soon as she settled down and I explained that this often happens. She said that Woody was moving his body into her hands and described a different kind of love from her normal affection for him. She knew that the healing was empowering her too and she believed totally in what she was doing.

I had warned her not to project sympathy onto Woody and she reported that the fear she had about his illness had disappeared. Her vulnerable mindset was no longer getting in the way as she surrendered to the belief that she could do it.

Woody, she told me, was getting very excited about food now. She had been observing him and had noticed how his eyes shone, how his ears pricked up at food time now. Not so long ago, he wouldn't get out of bed for the dried food but now she was giving him eggs, chickens and sardines, basmati rice, mince, liver and he was wolfing it all down. She had made friends with her butcher who she had never known was just down the road, and he was getting cheap cuts in especially for her dog. She told me that she had discovered that there's always a way round. If she couldn't find liver in her local convenience store, she was able to get it from the butcher now. This dog had lost pints of blood and even the vet was worried about the amount of steroids he was on. They may have been making him comfortable, but he was deteriorating quickly as a result. You don't keep a dog permanently on steroids; vets know this.

Over the next three months and after about half a dozen healings over the phone, the nose bleeds had completely stopped. But a couple of weeks later Woody had a relapse, so I invited my students and graduates to join me in a distant healing. The nosebleeds stopped again. Sally had given her permission for me to talk to them about his illness (something that is essential because of patient confidentiality) and she was overjoyed at the success.

I began training Sally in how to make her own meditative space and place Woody in the healing light herself. I also suggested that Woody should be kept at the family home until he was strong enough to cope with sleepovers at her husband's new home. He needed to be kept warm, to be fed regularly and not to be disorientated while he was in recovery.

A month later, Sally was healing him two or three times a week, and was already changing the way that she saw the world. From her self-doubt and fear of failure, she had evolved into a role model for the rest of the family, and even her estranged husband Johnny was becoming a more responsible father. It was clear that the chaos of the past was becoming organized, that Sally was taking on the position of being the leader of the pack, dealing with real emotions rather than papering over the cracks in the family's relationships.

It was her intention now to look after the entire family, including Woody, and to focus on taking responsibility for his health. She knew that she was healing herself. When you ground yourself, those scattered emotions and thoughts find a home, and Sally said that she had never felt stronger or more solid as a mother and a woman.

Woody is now completely recovered. Woody's family, too, have worked through a great deal of difficult issues. I was so glad that my students had also taken a part in this; such a total healing is very affirming.

> *When the vet said that if Woody lost a lot of blood again the best thing would be putting him to sleep, my family were devastated. All we could do was pray, pray for a miracle. After I spoke on the phone to Elizabeth, she said she was sending remote healing to Woody. Wow, within a short time his energy had changed, he was brighter and the spark was back in his eye. I tell you this: nothing beats the power of prayer and the power of pure love, and when a group of healers gets together anything is possible, anything. Elizabeth has a wonderful gift, she is truly blessed.*
> SALLY

On the Road

The travelling clinic is my opportunity to take my skills out to where they are needed. Most of the time it's just me, my car and my box of herbs and oils, and sometimes I'll be healing on the side of the road before I even get to my destination. I'll see a deer that has been hit by a car, or a rat dying by the side of the road, or even a rabbit with myxomatosis, and I'll be out with my bag like a shot to see what I can do.

Myxomatosis is a fatal disease introduced into the wild by humans to keep the wild rabbit population down. I see a great deal of it at the wildlife sanctuary where I work, which takes in wild rabbits, seagulls, foxes and other feral animals. Myxomatosis is an appalling disease and looks terrible, leaving the rabbit's eyes encrusted horribly. The rabbit's balance and coordination quickly deteriorate and it is barely able to breathe. Myxomatosis is widely regarded as incurable, but I have healed a number of rabbits. At the wildlife sanctuary I once used an aloe vera topical application to help a wild rabbit called Amber. I added a few drops of yarrow as an antibiotic and antiviral and gave her a pipette of rose hip tea. An animal can never be force-fed; even if it opens its mouth it will expel whatever it doesn't want, but Amber gently took the pipette. Her immune system was completely depleted, but with the help of the vitamin C from the rose hip she made a full recovery, much to everyone's amazement. I believe that it was the dedication of the centre manager in pipetting regularly that saved that rabbit's life. No one had ever heard of even a domestic rabbit recovering from myxomatosis, let alone a wild one.

I spend a lot of time working in rescue centres, and each visit is carefully planned and in my diary, but sometimes I get the nod about a van of animals being shipped over from one of the puppy or kitten farms, usually from Ireland. I get a text or email from my network of healers and rescue charities, and I down tools and head straight off to the port.

We arrive in various cars like something out of a TV cop show, swooping in to stop the van. Confronting the driver is the least of our challenges; while a couple of us stop the van, the others open the back doors and often find scores of pedigree pups and kittens with bones broken by the cramped conditions they have been transported in. Some have already been suffocated, literally squashed to death, while others have been sitting in their own excrement for the duration of the trip. Disorientated and blinded by the daylight after their short lives in cramped sheds, these pedigree pets are destined for the European market. It makes me shiver when

I see mobile phone numbers in the freebie papers advertising pups for sale, knowing that this is often the way that these poor little creatures are sold on. Some of my colleagues have gone undercover to find out more about this illegal trade and followed a phone call up with a clandestine meeting on a street corner or in a pub to find the pup under an arm or in a box.

Rescue Work

After my first visit as a trainee practitioner to the Brecon rescue centre and witnessing the effect on the animals there, it's hard to keep away from them these days. I felt so empowered by the knowledge that I could make a difference in the middle of such desperation and need that it became a defining moment in my career. I'm so grateful to Siobhan, her lovely pot-bellied pigs Lydia and Biddy, and Jake the rat for allowing me that opportunity when I had yet to graduate from my studies. Siobhan is one of those amazing people who have dedicated their lives to animals that have been abused and abandoned, and who have been so inspiring to me over the last ten years.

I made a point of making contact with some of my local rescue centres early on, and the work I do here is now built into my animal healing course so that my students get a chance to feel as inspired as I did. It's important that they feel grounded with their new skills, and there are few places more able to provide that experience than a rescue centre.

There are not enough hours in the day for me to do the work that I would like to do, but I'm careful to work with no more than four animals a day in my healing clinic, although at a rescue centre I may heal many more. On average an appointment lasts for an hour and a half and I often give the owners a healing during that time, and that becomes a long day.

I watch my students when they first arrive at a rescue centre, and see how much of a shock it is for them to be around so much pain. It's not just the animals who need the healing; the other care workers are often holding on to a lot of energy from the animals too, and the air can be thick with distress. I teach my students to protect themselves through the attunement process, and right from day one I've followed a strict routine myself. As much as you spread your stardust, you need to be fit, mentally, physically and emotionally, so that you can be a really good channel of that energy. You have to be a spiritual warrior.

I always allow myself plenty of time to get my kit together, packing my oils and herbs into my bags the night before and making sure that I take a bigger selection than I would normally use in the clinic. I also pack a camera so that I can photograph the rescue animals for our distant healing sessions. My travelling clinic is a much bigger operation, and I have to be prepared for all eventualities, and all weathers. Some of the bays are outside, so I often get drenched and need a change of clothes, or if I'm dealing with cats with FIV (feline immunodeficiency virus) and need to go into isolated units, I take Hibiscrub disinfectant with me in case the rescue centre has run out of its own supply. My clothes go straight into a hot wash when I get home to avoid me bringing anything nasty back to my clinic.

Many of these centres are a long way away and it's important that I spend five to ten minutes collecting my thoughts with a little meditation before going in. If I'm with my students, we will do it together and confirm our intention to heal as many animals as possible, to see them well, to be a good channel of energy and to spread a bit of happiness.

One of my favourite centres is the Celia Hammond Trust, nestled deep in a forest on the Sussex/Kent border. I always feel that I'm entering a meditation as I'm driving through. It's what England used to be like, with ancient oaks lining the little roads, far away from the noisy motorways that brought me there. The Trust is based in the grounds of a beautiful old house, with chalets dotted about outside. Most of the cats are allowed to roam freely. This is the ultimate in cat sanctuaries: a real cat heaven with a few cats in trees and others basking in the sunshine in the lovely gardens.

Corridors in the main cattery lead off into bedrooms for the cats and a beautiful lounge for the elderly cats, with hand-crocheted blankets on comfy old sofas. I always end up there at the end of the afternoon, sitting on a sofa and offering healing to these happy old cats. I am especially fond of Dudley, who has been there for years and who reminds me of General Melchett as played by Stephen Fry in *Blackadder Goes Forth*. He is the indisputable leader of the pack: even I feel I should stand to attention when I see him. Sadly he lost his ears to skin cancer, a common condition among feral and semi-feral cats who live and sleep outside. Even so, Dudley always responds well to the healing sessions.

Some of the feral cats with lighter-coloured skin use the room to shelter from the heat of the summer afternoons, and I apply my aloe vera topical lotion to their sunburn. I have yet to perfect a plant-based sunscreen.

Carolyn is an angel and a real leader of her team. She has built up good working relationships with other charities and organizations and become part of a network of like-minded souls whose mission is to help give a better life to animals in need. She believes in giving the best quality of life that she can offer them for as long as it takes. Her compassion is evident in all the workers here and is a wonderful example of my maxim that energy follows thought. She has been able to juggle successfully a lot of personalities here, and clearly brings a good deal of happiness to a lot of people and animals. She knows how to make decisions that would make me collapse in a heap because she is so together and so grounded. There are no ego trips at this centre. Carolyn knows that it is not about her, and from that realization her work appears effortless.

Most of their work involves rescuing stray or abandoned cats after a tip-off by phone from somebody who has found a litter of kittens under a shed or at a caravan park or a building site. Some come to them after an elderly or ill owner has died, and they don't discriminate against any cats. Most are successfully re-homed, and the Trust is rigorous about vetting potential new homes. In the case of feral cats, they are put out to work as a more humane solution to rat infestations than some of the poisons on the market; unlike a domestic cat, a feral cat's response to a rat is instinctive and Carolyn helps to re-home them to smallholdings, stables and farms as a deterrent to rodents. Smallholders have told her that mice and rats have moved out since the cats' arrival.

My own dogs, Lily and Morris, came from two independent rescue centres. I was very impressed with the strict guidelines placed on my home and work environment by these rescue centres, and how they insisted that my dogs not be left alone all day and that they get plenty of exercise. I am always impressed how much knowledge these charity workers have about a particular animal and what type of set-up would suit it best. They understand animals' individual needs and really care about their long-term wellbeing. It is a big responsibility to care for another being; I believe that it's a privilege rather than a right to own an animal, and no one understands this more clearly than rescue workers.

My job as a healer when I visit a rescue centre is to enhance the animals' quality of life. Many strays have had very little human contact and enjoy the deeply relaxing healing session that my students, graduates and I can offer them. We do hands-off healing if they prefer not to have their space invaded, as well as hands-on healing and lots of play with the kittens. At Celia Hammond, 'cuddle carers' come in every day to provide some light to the grief-stricken or lonely cats. I'll admit that I do leave there sometimes wishing I could give them a home, but my menagerie of eight animals is already a full-time job in itself. My fellow healing students and graduates feel the same way, and many have extended that lifeline by offering a home to many of the animals they have healed, from rabbits to cats, ferrets to dogs.

Sometimes I don't know what's going to happen to the cats I've just been healing, but there is a point where I have to leave it all behind. I feel worrying about the unexpected is not going to help anybody, and so I quickly change my thoughts to visualize that animal settled in a good, loving home.

I feel totally absorbed in the place while I'm there, but I have to be content to do what I can. With most of my animal patients I have the opportunity to forge a relationship over time, but at a rescue centre I often only get one chance to see an animal before it is re-homed or passes away, and the animals usually need so many levels of healing. Like us, every animal is different and sometimes it takes a few sessions to deeply access an animal. Occasionally it will let me in on that first and only meeting. That is a tremendous privilege.

I believe that we should all consider offering a rescue dog or cat a good home before looking at alternatives. At Celia Hammond, as with many other rescue centres, all the cats have been assessed, neutered, microchipped, wormed, flea-treated and vaccinated. Some rescue centres even offer free insurance. They have lots of advice and are usually better informed than a private seller about which animal will suit a particular home environment.

Michelle and Ollie

Sometimes I see animals that have been brought back to a rescue centre again and again after their new owners have underestimated the reality of living with a rescued pet. Ollie was a six-year-old Corgi/Alsatian cross when Michelle re-homed her from a rescue centre in Sussex. The poor thing had already been re-homed seven times over two years because of mismanaged placements; despite being described as aggressive she had been repeatedly placed with children, so it was little surprise when she was returned again and again to the rescue charity. As a result, Ollie was utterly disconnected from the world around her, and when Michelle finally gave her a home she couldn't even walk on a lead. She didn't recognize her name and tried to run away when Michelle tried to touch her.

Michelle works full time, so her mother Josie took on the role of being Ollie's main carer during the day. As Josie had a lovely dog herself, called Murphy, Michelle thought that some of Ollie's behaviour issues might be eased by the new relationship. Most rescue dogs come with very little history, and very often details of their puppyhood will never be available to their new owners. Puppies must be kept with their siblings and their mother for at least eight weeks for many good reasons, not least for the socialization that goes on within the pack. Puppies learn many of their basic skills at this age, and it was clear that Ollie had been deprived of these too early. At six years old she was still not completely toilet trained and felt insecure and dominated by Josie's dog Murphy. She could not relax, catnapping instead of sleeping, and barking constantly if Michelle or Josie left her alone with only Murphy for company. She seemed unable to live comfortably in her new surroundings, bumping into the glass patio door again and again as if, each time, she was coming across it for the first time.

Dog-training classes didn't solve the problem and Michelle was asked to leave the class. She tried behaviour therapy and even asked the vet to check out Ollie's mental state, before a recommendation from my local pet shop owner, Leanne, brought her to me. I had helped Leanne with two hyperactive rescue dogs in the past who, after four healings, had become well grounded and much more socialized.

The first time she came to the clinic, Ollie squatted down and used my lovely rug as her makeshift toilet, much to Michelle's embarrassment. I could see how nerve-racking it was for Michelle to second-guess how Ollie was going to behave away from home; she was like a cat on hot bricks at first. I concentrated on putting Michelle at ease. The mess on my rug was not important; I quickly cleared it up and got straight down to work.

Michelle had a wonderfully compassionate nature and soon opened her mind to the kind of work that I do. I asked Michelle to offer Ollie the oils, and Ollie walked away after sniffing deeply at the violet leaf (helpful for past trauma and stress). This is often a sign that an oil has hit a nerve, and we watched as Ollie processed it, licking and chewing for a while, then walking back for more. Michelle offered her the calendula too, and this time Ollie grabbed hold of the bottle in her mouth and licked the oil out of Michelle's hand.

She was only interested in the violet leaf and calendula, and so I put the box of oils away and settled into the healing. Ollie and Michelle relaxed deeply, both sighing gently. By the end of the session, it was as if two new beings stood up to leave. Michelle told me that she had never felt so relaxed. She could not get over how focused Ollie was; she had always seemed so chaotic, Michelle told me, yet now she was calm, relaxed and present. (Michelle told me later that when she went to her kick-boxing class the next evening, nobody could move her, she was so solid and grounded!)

After the healing, Ollie behaved like a 'normal dog' for a full three weeks before going downhill again. Suddenly she would howl, scratching the carpet and peeing around the house. This is a typical healing crisis, and often happens when the first level has been peeled back enough for the real work to begin. Michelle booked Ollie back in immediately, and this time when I offered her the rose oil, she was ready to start to open up. Rose works on a very deep level, and for many animals suffering deep trauma, it's too much if offered too soon. They can only go there when they are ready.

Michelle had seen the difference after the first session and was totally committed to seeing Ollie through the next few weeks. As Ollie gradually began to calm down, Michelle also started to relax more. She was fascinated by the healing and was one of the first people to sign up for my diploma in animal healing. She and Ollie came regularly to the monthly healing meditation evenings, and we soon became friends.

As she spent more and more time at the clinic, helping out with my animals, harvesting the herbs with me, studying how I make up the oils and heal my own animals, she realized that she was swapping the intense pressure of city work for a more rural, relaxed way of being. Her stressful lifestyle was finding a better balance, making her work life much more bearable. She began to use creative meditations and positive affirmations to help her get through the day, and to enhance the quality of her work and her life. She learned how to put boundaries down, how to leave work in the office and get back in time to take Ollie for a lovely long walk. The happier she became, the more content her beautiful dog became.

While Michelle was changing her life, Ollie, now quite an old lady, had developed senile dementia and was deteriorating very quickly. She could no longer walk without falling over and had lost a lot of her cognitive skills. The vet suggested putting her down, but Michelle couldn't let go yet. She brought her over to see if there was anything I could do to make Ollie's quality of life better, and we conducted a beautiful healing together. Neither of us was surprised when, after the healing, Ollie got up and wandered around the room before going out to play with Lily in the garden. This had felt like a dynamic double act of energy. I felt so proud to be healing with this woman, who had shown such commitment both to herself and to her dog over the years that we had known each other.

Some time later, Michelle confided that she had been getting a lot of pressure from her family to put Ollie down, but after this wonderful session she had found the courage to say no. This was the first time she had ever stood up to her parents and put her point across clearly, and yet she did it so passionately that they agreed to support her plan to monitor Ollie carefully on a day-to-day basis, to take each day as it came. She felt that Ollie would know when it was her time to go. Michelle had taken charge of what she believed to be right, and her parents, although shocked at her conviction, respected her for making her decision.

Within two weeks Ollie was better than she had been for months and, with regular healings, she lived for another year before she finally died of kidney failure at the ripe old age of 13. Nobody, not least the vet, could believe her fabulous longevity.

Ollie had put Michelle on the path to where she is now, and that is a great gift. Seven months after Ollie passed away, Michelle felt ready to give a home to Archie, a beautiful six-month-old schnauzer cross who already seems to have healing abilities of his own. Michelle's mother was recently diagnosed with a cancerous growth on her foot and is undergoing chemotherapy, but Michelle says that Archie often licks this foot and rests his head on it. Trials have been conducted on dogs who have been used to sniff out cancer in humans; I'm fascinated to see the outcome of this.

Many of my clients have been so impressed with the effect of healing on their pets that they have done my animal healing course, but Michelle is the one who has really followed in my footsteps. Like Wow did with me, Ollie led her to change her life, to reassess her work/play balance and to immerse herself in a new world of knowledge and understanding. She has also done the animal aromatics course and graduated from the diploma in equine healing with me, and is now embarking on an animal behaviour degree with the intention of setting up her own practice in her new home.

In the meantime, the legacy of Ollie is already finding a place in Michelle's own animal healing clinic. Thanks to her, Michelle now truly knows who she is and has the confidence to do what she really believes in. I reckon that there will be a lot of animals and their owners who will be deeply indebted to Ollie over the next few years.

> The healing sessions with Elizabeth helped to create a strong bond between myself and Ollie. They also helped Ollie to be more balanced and behave like a 'normal dog'. I feel the healing course was the first steps of my healing journey. I am very grateful for the experience and look forward to wherever it may take me.
> MICHELLE

Bat Rescue

> Liz's attention to correct nutrition and her relaxed manner with animals are compatible with the rehabilitation of delicate, sensitive animals like bats. Remember, however, that bats should not be handled without first getting advice from the Bat Conservation Trust.
> BAT HOSPITAL, SUSSEX

As my network of students grows, I am so excited about spreading the word about healing around the world. My days are filled with meeting astonishing people who often change their lives to work with animals, as Michelle did. So it's always such a joy when I meet someone who changes *my* world, whose commitment and knowledge open up a whole new chapter for me.

I met Amanda through one of the smallest animals I have ever worked with.

I heal all sorts of animals, from dogs to donkeys, cats to tigers, rats to snakes, but when Brian brought me a bat which he had found dying at the end of the drive one Sunday afternoon while I was teaching my students, it was so tiny that I wondered if I could make a difference.

Brian had already put it in a cardboard box and, after the students had gone, I pulled the curtains shut so that it would be as dark as the bat's natural environment and put it on my lap. Mia, one of my advanced animal healing students, stayed behind to help me. I began to attune immediately as his little body was already so cold and I could feel the life force slipping away.

I felt sure that this was male energy; after being around so many budgies and other birds, tortoises, snakes and other animals over the last ten years, I really can tell the difference between male and female energy. I put my hands close to his tiny body and he soaked up the healing, his ears uncurling and standing right up. I didn't know at the time, but this was a long-eared bat, or a whispering bat as it is sometimes known. He was clearly responding to the energy in my hands. As I scanned his body, I intuitively felt drawn to healing his left radius, which was absorbing more energy. I was sure that he had broken it.

After half an hour's healing I rang Reg, my ornithologist friend, and told him that I needed help. I had warmed up the bat's little body, but I didn't have a clue how to rehabilitate him. I had a vague idea that bats most probably ate gnats and insects, but how would I feed them to him?

Reg happened to have the number of a local woman who rescues bats and I got straight on the phone. As she was only up the road, I hopped in the car and drove over with Mia. While she drove, I held the bat, whom I called Aaron, in my hands, feeling sure that the heat from my hands was keeping him alive. Some bats can carry rabies but somehow I knew he wouldn't bite me. I was sending him messages of support throughout the short journey, and I felt he knew that my intentions were pure.

When we arrived, Mia and I couldn't believe what an amazing world we had stepped into. This was straight out of *The Good Life*, with ducks and chickens and their proud cockerel waddling freely around a garden bursting with smells, colour and life. The kind of herbs that grew there were those that I have tried (and failed) to grow and I sniffed enviously at the marshmallow, which is great for upper respiratory tract issues, as well as valerian, lady's mantle and lemongrass.

Amanda came to the door, her beautiful blond hair scraped back in a bun revealing the face of an angel. She took Aaron from me and had a good look as we walked into her clinic, and quickly confirmed that he was male and that he had indeed broken his left radius. She was concerned that he might not see the night through, but was fascinated by how relaxed he seemed to be, and I told her a little about the healing I had been doing.

As I do with my new patients, Amanda did a consultation and I told her what I could. She picked out a clean paintbrush from a pot and dipped it into a glass of water, put it to his mouth and, after a moment, he began to suck. This was so magical to watch for me; I never cease to be amazed at the dedication and understanding of some of the amazing people I meet on my travels.

She then opened a drawer in her clinic and revealed hundreds of wriggling mealworms, which she feeds on porridge oats and carrots before feeding to her bats. Picking one up with a tweezer, she offered it to Aaron – who devoured it in one. I quickly sent healing to the mealworms before they disappeared! I hate watching animals eat others alive; when I'm with bearded dragons, which eat locusts, I often don't know where to look!

Aaron got through the night, and when I came back the next day I was thrilled to see that he had had a good healthy poo. A good poo is always the sign of a healthy animal, and this was firm, with no blood in it, which showed me that there was no internal damage. He was fast asleep, hanging upside down, and I gently did another healing. As soon as I attuned to him, his ears fluttered up again. It felt like he knew it was me.

Amanda had another single male who needed a companion, and she suggested that when he was completely rehabilitated, Aaron would stay with him. As I looked around, I did healings on some of the other bats, and tuned in to the amazing energy of this wonderful place. Although Amanda's priority is to release the bats, some are too badly hurt and instead accompany her (once they are back in full health) on her educational talks. Amanda spends a lot of time organizing talks about the serious decline of bats due to the destruction of their natural habitats. Pesticides are one of the biggest problems for them. They are protected, but they are so unpopular that most people are unlikely to call the helpline if they find one that needs help.

Amanda walked me back to the car and I asked her about her fabulous garden. She told me a little about the eco-system that she has created there, and how much of it is designed around her honey. She is an extremely successful bee-keeper, and her honey recently came second in the South of England show.

I lusted after the beehives that lined the back garden, their residents happily collecting the pollen from the profusion of flowers and herbs. This was sensational. Traditional bee-keepers like Amanda are very worried about the mass production of bee-keeping. In the US it's already very worrying because hives are often piled on trucks and moved to a different region so that the bees can produce a speciality orange blossom or almond blossom, premium products these days for the supermarkets. Once they have harvested the pollen there, they are moved on. Imagine the stress the bees have to endure when they are locked into their hives for a whole day of travelling, and yet they still manage to produce such a magical medicinal food: manuka honey, the queen bee of honeys, well known for its antibacterial and antibiotic properties. It is now being tested in hospitals and by cancer research groups.

Amanda and I discussed how bees know instinctively what to bring back to the hive to keep it healthy, and that all bee-keepers should be growing medicinal plants to help them. Infection can sweep through whole colonies; Amanda uses thyme, an antibacterial herb, with garlic cloves in her beehives to keep her bees healthy. I have been observing bees for some time and noting what medicinal plants they head for, and I was pleased to hear Amanda had the same plants growing in her garden that I had listed.

Amanda showed me how they feast on her borage, and I could see their little legs packed with the brilliant blue pollen. She also grows echinacea, with its beautiful purple flowers. Echinacea is brimming with energy and packed with antibacterial, antiviral properties, and is an immuno-stimulant and antimicrobial – all of which the bees know well.

I've noted that it is the brightly coloured vegetables and plants that are, as a rule, the best medicinal plants, and bees always head straight for the most beautiful vibrant reds and oranges of marjoram and calendula, the indigo of phacelia, and all the feel-good, high-vibrational colours of the garden.

I asked Amanda if I could come and meditate with the bees. It was such a glorious vision, this garden, and I am so worried about the millions of bees who are dying around the world. I wanted to be around them so I could understand a little more while I am distant-healing. Amanda graciously agreed and we arranged a date before she sent me home with a dozen eggs from her fabulous chickens and several jars of honey to use in my home-made dog and cat biscuits. It was so lovely for me to see so many healthy, happy animals. She even gave me a wild rabbit to release into the wild. She was healing the healer.

Synchronicity

*By way of the beehive the whole cosmos enters man
and makes him strong and able.*
RUDOLPH STEINER

As far as I can see, over this extraordinary journey of the last ten years, what goes around does tend to come around. My intention is always to do the highest good, to be a channel for the purest form of healing, and I notice that the more work I do, the more the universe supports me.

I know I'm not alone; synchronicity, the growing number of inexplicable coincidences which many people on a spiritual journey experience, confirms that the universe really does provide. For me it's a lovely reminder of the growing connection I feel as I continue to expand the intuitive part of my mind. It's rather handy most of the time, too. On many occasions it's an animal who brings me into contact with what I need most, however random it may seem at the time.

Helen and Felix

I met Helen at a talk I was doing on animal healing at a complementary health clinic in Brighton some years ago. I had taken time out from making my latest meditation CD to do this; I love making music and find it very relaxing, but we had come across a musical block and I needed to get out of the studio for a while. My sister Susie and I had been making a particularly angelic piece of music and decided that we needed a soprano to sing the role of the archangel. We had emailed and phoned our network to find someone but, so far, every route had come to a dead end. The workshop was a great way to unwind and think about something else.

There were only half a dozen people at the workshop but it was a lovely group. Every one of the group was fascinated by animal healing, but Helen caught my eye immediately. She was very beautiful but absolutely tiny. She reminded me of a delicate little sparrow. She was very quiet but utterly focused throughout the session, and after the two hours she took me aside to ask if I would do a private consultation on her cat, Felix, who was having territorial problems with the other neighbourhood cats. They had recently moved to a new house and Felix was fearful of going out. He had been a typical tom and had loved sloping off at night, but since the move he had lost his confidence and stayed inside all the time.

Felix also hated travelling in the car, so I agreed to go to Helen's house the following week. When I arrived, Helen's father came to the door. He was a very imposing figure and I felt like a little girl going to see her best friend as he ushered me into the sitting room. The feeling didn't last, though, once I spotted the baby grand piano amid a stack of music scores and a well-used music stand. Perhaps this was the introduction to a musical network that would lead me to my soprano!

Helen and Felix were waiting for me in the sitting room and, as I greeted them, I asked who played the piano. She said that she did, but her real love was singing. I didn't say anything, but I made a mental note of yet another coincidence confirming that I was in the right place. We sat down and, as I reached into my bag for a consultation form, I casually asked what kind of singing she was into. When she told me that she was a freelance soprano, my heart began to pound. I love these kinds of moments, but I didn't feel that I could launch into my musical needs. The world of classical music is a world away from meditation CDs, and it would take a very special person to be able to leap from one to the other. Besides, this was Felix's time, so I put the thought away and completely focused on him.

Felix, a beautiful tortoiseshell tabby, was rubbing himself up against me, much to Helen's surprise as he had been so fearful of any new people since they had moved. I always attune in the car before I go into a new house to ground myself after the travelling and to get the intention clear about what I am going to do. Felix seemed to be picking up on my calmer energy, purring and rubbing at my legs and sniffing at my box of oils. I laughed at myself as his tail reminded me of a conductor waving his baton.

Cats tend to sniff rather than lick the oils, and Felix was clearly choosing the violet leaf. He liked the chickweed but refused all the others, so I focused on his need for confidence as I began the healing. I lay on the carpet, placing my hands close to his body as his purring got louder and more rhythmic. He loved this. He began to extend his nails, clawing the carpet and rolling over, totally relaxed as I worked on him. It was as if he knew he could trust me to do what was needed.

Afterwards, Helen made me a cup of tea and we chatted about Felix and his confidence issues. She and Felix had moved back in with her parents while she began to travel around Europe with the opera company. She needed to save money and have someone to look after Felix while she was away, but she told me how this was a double-edged sword: her parents had made it possible for her to progress her career, but her father, who had also been a professional singer, was very protective about the choices she made.

There is a lot of rejection in Helen's world; she had already had some wonderful breaks and sung at prestigious venues, but she knew that the highs come with the lows and had dusted herself down on many occasions. She felt increasingly demoralized as she went up for auditions and was sometimes passed over for someone with more presence. She was worried that she was losing her nerve completely. She had even started speech and drama classes to build up her confidence. For such a tiny woman, she needed more than just a good voice to make it on stage. It occurred to me that Felix's confidence issues were a mirror to his mistress's.

As we chatted over our tea, Helen confessed that she was interested in a more spiritual journey than her parents approved of. She had done lots of singing in church and had a lovely ethereal energy around her, but she wasn't interested in traditional religion. Instead she was fascinated by what was happening with Felix and wanted to know more. She asked if she could come to me for some coaching; what I had told her about personal development had resonated with her. Many people are fascinated after a consultation with their animals. They witness the positive effects on their animals, but also recognize how good they feel, too. Naturally enough, they want to know more.

I sensed that Helen needed to break away from the mental confines of her family's expectations. Our parents may want the best for us, but it's essential for our self-esteem that we make our own way. A thought began to develop in my mind and I wondered how to broach the subject of her singing on my CD.

When she arrived for her coaching, I asked her how Felix was and she told me that she was thrilled how confident he had become in the garden. She confessed that she had been in two minds about whether to come or not, but when Felix had started going out again almost immediately after the healing, and seemed to own his space, she was intrigued.

We headed into the clinic to begin her session and she passed some of my meditation CDs piled high on my table ready to be packed up and sent out. She asked me about them and I found myself tongue-tied for a moment. My music is very contemporary, more like film music than classical. Some people need music to help them focus on their meditation and I like to use natural sounds as much as possible. I told her about my owl meditation featuring the call of five British breeds of owl including tawny, barn and little owl, which transports the listener into a night-time landscape. I didn't know if Helen would laugh at me or be embarrassed if I asked her if she would sing the archangel role on the CD, but I bit the bullet and asked her if could play the music to her and, if she liked it, if she would consider singing on it.

I showed Helen the lyrics that my sister had written and played the track, and although I don't think she had heard anything like it before, she loved it. The music is very ethereal and the lyrics are beautifully poetic and, to my amazement, she began to sing along, a huge, powerful, angelic voice emanating from her tiny frame. She was perfect.

For Helen to do something like this, allowing her own musicality to guide her rather than a piece of sheet music, was stretching for her. Her classical training had not allowed her this amount of freedom before and she didn't know quite what to do with it at first. But she had witnessed her cat overcoming his confidence problems, and had obviously decided to give it a go herself.

The resulting CD is fabulous. Helen was finally singing to her own tune and getting tremendous confidence from it. And what's so lovely is that the synchronicity continues. I didn't just get what I needed; work for her is pouring in now that Helen has opened this door into a new realm. She has changed her way of thinking and the universe is littering her with rewards. It's been an amazing journey from an animal healing workshop to where she is now in her career, and I love to think that Felix was a facilitator in her spiritual growth.

International Rescue

We're a nation of animal lovers in the UK and our cultural values are not always shared around the world. It's hard not to make judgements when you see how some animals are kept, even as near as in southern Europe, but this is a world in which dogs are kept to hunt, cats to rat and where donkeys are still beasts of burden. Animals are treated as workers rather than the pets they would be in this country, and dogs and cats usually live outside. Old, arthritic animals who are no longer useful, or kittens and puppies without homes to go to, are often left to fend for themselves. It breaks my heart to see the scores of dead animals on fast roads. I'll always stop the car and pick up a dead cat in the road and, out of respect for its dignity, gently lay it in the hedge and say a little prayer for it before heading on my way.

Despite the difference in attitude, or maybe because of it, I've always been fascinated by other cultures. I would love to travel more and share with locals how healing can benefit all animals. Since my early twenties I have searched out the kind of holidays that support local environmental issues, particularly in places where the tourist industry could otherwise endanger the local wildlife. It's a great way to meet local people, as well as like-minded holidaymakers. I went on a bee study on the Mayan Peninsula with local Mexicans some years ago, and learned so much about the country and the people, as well as the impact of bees on the planet. We hear about the destruction of the rainforests all the time these days, but seeing first-hand the effect that this has on the parrots and all the other wildlife whose homes have been destroyed can make you rethink the way you live in the world.

Environmental tourism encourages governments to protect natural habitats, such as in Tobago where turtles lay their eggs in the sand in the early hours of the morning, and proves that there is money to be made from conservation holidays. Tobago takes its turtles very seriously now.

I find that the more you find out what's going on in the world, the more involved you feel. I feel so much better being connected to the local culture than I do when I'm just lying around a pool. As soon as I arrive on holiday, I ask at my hotel where the nearest rescue centre or sanctuary is so that I can go and give my support, even if it's just a donation. It might take a while to find out, but it's always worth it because I meet so many great people along the way.

A few years after I had set up the clinic, it occurred to me that instead of giving donations I could give my time to rescue centres in places like Spain, Portugal, Morocco and Cyprus. I set up The Healing Animals Organisation to build an international network of vets, sanctuaries and healers to work together. As my student healers graduate with their diploma in animal healing, I hope that our work will spread its tentacles even more widely.

These days, news of my work travels quickly and I am often invited to travel to rescue centres in southern Europe which provide a safe haven for animals turned out by farmers who no longer want the responsibility of an older cat with increasing vet bills. There may be nothing wrong with the cat, and the owner may have fed and loved that cat for the last ten years or more, but cats are considered workers, and many farmers simply trade them in for a younger model when they stop catching mice as well as they once did. At least these farmers bring the cats into the sanctuary where they can be looked after.

Cyprus

Brian thought that we might be able to snatch a little 'us' time when we booked a five-day trip to Cyprus, but I think as soon as he saw just how many animals I could help at the British-run sanctuaries I had tracked down, he knew where my priorities would lie and resigned himself to driving me around the island in the intense heat instead. He's a marvellous man and understands just how important my work is to me. He is a real animal lover himself and, from the moment we walked in, I didn't even need to explain where we would be spending the next five days. It was a sanctuary located in the middle of a UN buffer zone at what was once Nicosia airport. Until the Turks invaded in 1974, it had been Cyprus's international airport; one can only imagine the fear and anxiety when everyone had had to drop everything and leave. A 747 passenger plane still sits on the landing strip as a reminder of how time stopped for hundreds of thousands of locals, who became refugees overnight.

As we drove up to the gates of the sanctuary, I felt like I was in a time warp. It was all so quiet and empty, and felt eerily like a film set. The place is only 200 miles from Lebanon, 400 miles from Israel and 40 miles from Turkey, so it's right in the middle of a hot spot, and the combination of the strange silence and the knowledge of so much suffering, both past and present, gave my visit extra poignancy.

The dog shelter is right in the middle of all this, run for the last 15 years by an amazing woman called Sharon whose husband works for the United Nations. He is currently in Afghanistan and is usually jetting around the world on UN business, so Sharon is able to pour her heart and soul into her work at the shelter.

There are a couple of makeshift rooms and an amazing array of donated stainless-steel tables. The place is immaculate, which is amazing considering how dependent she is on donations. I knew that they couldn't afford medication and were desperate for help, and phoned to offer my services. For me, it is about shovelling poo just as much as showing them how to use indigenous plant materials to save themselves a fortune. She readily accepted.

Sharon runs the sanctuary almost single-handed with just brother-and-sister team Dan and Sundun to help. Dan and Sundun have fled their home in Sri Lanka because of the troubles there. It was so peaceful being there with them; these beautiful people had lost half their family and yet they were so open to healing animals. Dan told me that he would love to come and train with me, but that he couldn't leave this place with the 200 dogs and 50 pups. Sharon, too, is exceptionally generous and has never refused a dog, although she does have a euthanasia policy and is very realistic about what she can do for them.

It's a fabulous place where dogs roam in large packs. They have pens for the night, but there are no boundaries by day, and it's lovely to see them basking in the sunshine. You only have to look at their behaviour to see how happy they are. Obviously they do get the odd troublemaker, but Sharon, Dan and Sundun are experienced enough now to spot a dog who has been mentally or physically abused and who may be tricky in the pack. Sharon told me about a Rottweiler that had been trained as a guard dog and was terrifying at first. Sharon wondered how she would get him out of the van when he first arrived. Eventually, she used a piece of meat to lure him away and he was kept well away from the others until he was rehabilitated. It's all based on common sense.

As soon as I started working with the animals, the effect on them was clear. Even Sharon's guard dogs sniffed me, wagging their tails happily. It's impossible to have a placebo effect with animals, and the calm and trust that comes out of the work is immediate. I knew that my time there was precious as soon as I started to work with this incredibly dedicated team, and we all had a real knowledge that something quite special was happening.

We got organized. We divided the dogs into the two rooms, one for the puppies and one for the older dogs. One person would go to the kennel and get a dog while I would swab another down with a special tick-and-flea treatment wash of aloe vera base with small quantities of tea tree, lavender and German chamomile. Although I knew that I would have a conveyor belt of puppies coming through, my intention was to heal each individual dog as I was washing it.

Dan and Sundun pray as part of their practice, and so they were grounded and focused, totally present. There was no shouting, just pure dedicated silence. Dan had worried that it would be chaotic to do all the puppies in one session, but I asked him to visualize it going well. And it went like clockwork. Dan and Sundun couldn't believe how the puppies were enjoying this 'spa treatment'. Dan and Sundun thought I had to be a holy person, because the puppies would normally squeal and fidget while being swabbed. These were abandoned, hungry pups, many of whom were suffering from diarrhoea, yet all was beautifully hushed in the clinic.

Dan and Sundun could be great healers. They were so empty of ego, such gorgeous souls. If energy follows thought, it was because of *their* energy that this place was so peaceful. It was like walking into a place of worship, even if the dogs were barking outside. The mindset is everything: if every thought comes from the heart, miracles can happen.

After the tick-and-flea wash, we went outside and worked on Libby, a beautiful Cyprus poodle whose front legs had been deliberately run over by some young joyriders. Her legs were in splints and I really did have to hold myself together as I offered her the oils. She licked the violet leaf (useful for fear and new surroundings) and calendula (for deep emotional issues), deeply inhaling the rose (for physical and emotional trauma). Libby then took the comfrey macerated oil (for broken bones) and the seaweed oil (a natural electrolyte). She must have been terribly hot in those splints in the intense heat.

I do have a larger repertoire of oils, but I keep it very simple when I'm away; most of the issues in rescue centres are to do with deep psychological pain, separation and loss. Libby wagged her tail gently; I think she was pleased that someone was making a fuss of her. Sharon and her team had contained her in a nice pen with a cool breeze, but she needed something so much deeper.

We went on to see another Cyprus poodle called Becky, who had recently had six pups, only three of which had survived. She was terribly skinny, yet the pups were still suckling. Sharon told me that she had had problems feeding her, and there was still a bowl of uneaten dried food beside her. This lovely mother dog declined even a sniff of any of the oils. She didn't even want to go near them. She knew that they would get through to the milk for her pups, and she put their needs before her own. Sharon had never heard of this before and was amazed to see how instinctive animals are.

I put some sardines down for Becky and she weakly inched forward and began to eat. She was so appreciative, wagging her tail gently while taking in tiny amounts to avoid being sick. Brian and I had collected our leftovers from our hotel meals to take to the sanctuary. I'd even had a chat with the chef, who was marvellous and gave us leftover chicken and lamb to take to the dogs. I had all the dogs following me around, sniffing at my bag. One of them even stole my make-up bag, presumably in the hope that my lipstick and mascara might be as delicious as everything else in my handbag.

The puppies were drinking from Becky now and as she looked up at me with her sad eyes, I felt that she was thanking me. I reached over to heal the pups and she gently nosed them towards me, one by one. They were so tiny, only a few days old, and it was a joy to watch this maternal instinct in such desperate circumstances. Even Brian, who was in the room too, was speechless.

Sharon was so grateful for all this healing, and she and the Sri Lankan siblings were eager to find out how they could heal the dogs themselves after I had gone. I promised to teach Dan when I next come back and he was thrilled. He felt that he had been recognized. I feel sure that my visit there was the first of many, and that Dan will become a great healer.

Portugal

I am often invited to work with a wonderful vet called Miguel who rehabilitates donkeys in northern Portugal and specializes in the Miranda breed. The Miranda is a beautiful rich bay with long ears, a tough breed and larger than most species of donkey. I was there with one of my graduate healers from Lisbon who speaks English and Portuguese fluently, conducting healing sessions at Miguel's sanctuary and accompanying him on his home visits.

The locals in the area are mostly elderly, semi-retired and on low incomes. They have limited access to basic donkey care such as a farriers, equine dentists or vets. One of my jobs on that particular trip was to source local indigenous plant materials that could be used as forage for the many donkeys with badly cracked hooves, dull coats and spasmodic colic due to eating a diet of straw.

Surrounded by mountains, ravines and free-flowing streams, the raw beauty of this most northern part of Portugal took my breath away. As we drove through the windy roads, I asked Miguel to pull the car over so I could look at a sprawling mass of green plant growing on the riverbank and in the river itself. On closer inspection I realized that it was chickweed, a highly nutritious, safe medicinal plant which humans and animals alike have been eating for centuries. I chewed a little. It tasted like grass and was completely different to the spinach-like vegetable that I cook in a little butter at home. I carefully bagged up several handfuls to take back to the donkeys, while Miguel assured me that this plant grew everywhere and that we were not depleting precious stock.

As we headed off along the mountain path towards our next home visit, I spotted some beautiful old stone hedgerows with an abundance of wild roses sprawling through the thickets. My four horses forage up to 30 per cent of their time from the hedgerows at home, and love rose hips. Although this was the wrong time of the year for the hips, all parts of the rose are edible and I asked Miguel to pull over so that we could prune some of the stems and the lovely, dark green leaves, which are so nutritious and so wonderful for digestive-tract inflammation.

As we arrived at the smallholding I prepared myself for the healing session, breathing in the beauty of the countryside we had just driven through and attuning to the donkey, whose skin problems I was here to treat. I rummaged in my bag for the chickweed and offered it to her. She clearly loved it and devoured the lot, nosing in my bag for more. I carefully handed her the rose stems and, again, she adored them, nibbling at the leaves and stems. As she munched away I brought out some dried rose hips that I had brought from home and, again, she munched on them happily. Neither Miguel nor the donkey's owner had ever thought about tapping into the abundant local plant life for their animals, but were thrilled to realize that they would be able to collect chickweed and rose throughout the year.

We said our goodbyes to Miguel and headed off to the other end of the country. A 14-hour drive lay ahead of us, stopping in Lisbon overnight before heading into the hills of southern Portugal to meet an Englishman called Peter who had set up a donkey sanctuary when he and his partner had retired some years ago. After witnessing what often happens to these gorgeous animals when *they* are retired, Peter had bought a piece of land and a small farm to care for them.

There is no equivalent of the RSPCA in Portugal; animals who have outlived their use on the land are all too often left to their own devices. Donkeys are used as machinery on the farms and have been for working in the region for centuries. They are so loyal and hard working, but it's very expensive for farmers to keep looking after them in old age. With the advances of modern machinery and subsidies from the European Union, most farmers in this region no longer need donkeys at all. It is expensive to transport an old donkey to the nearest vet, and most farmers simply don't prioritize this. Even the abattoir is often too far for most farmers and, again, the cost of transportation is often considered not to be worthwhile when turning a donkey out to pasture naturally is seen as a perfectly acceptable alternative.

The sanctuary soon also became home to countless dogs and cats, malnourished, neglected and suffering from broken bones. Most animals are not spayed or neutered in southern Mediterranean countries, and there are simply too many for the country to cope with. Peter's wonderful vet comes from Germany to spay as many as they can a few times a year, but it is an insurmountable problem and it's not unusual for

Peter to receive a phone call about an abandoned cat with nine kittens.

We're not squeaky clean in the UK, either: farmers are not charities and they don't keep old animals who are no longer producing young or who are suitable for meat. Some are kept as surrogates or companions, but the majority are put down once their work is done.

Good animal husbandry is about looking after the needs of working animals, and an abattoir is a better option in my opinion than leaving an old animal to fend for itself when its day is done. Keeping a distressed animal alive with nobody taking responsibility for its welfare is terribly cruel.

I spoke to Peter at length on the phone from England to find out what kind of conditions the animals were suffering from and what I should bring with me. He was fascinated with how spiritual healing could help traumatized animals to relax and also by the work I had done in zoopharmacognosy. We talked about plants for hours as he began to see how they could heal their animals while keeping costs down. Peter had been a sheep farmer in Scotland for years and he knew his plants. He had also observed his animals self-selecting, as most good farmers will do, and he was very keen for me to come and set up a mini-apothecary for him to use there.

Peter and his team raise funds through second-hand furniture shops in the nearby town. With so many ex-pats making a second home for themselves, they make an adequate income for the sanctuary while finding potential animal-adopters at the same time. It is a tough business trying to re-home the many abandoned animals, however, and Peter had reached saturation point.

The majority of cats and dogs are re-homed to locals. This year alone Peter has re-homed 160 dogs and 80 cats under a strict vetting policy in which he does not sell any animals, relying only on donations so that he can find the right home. With Portuguese, Germans, Swedes and British in the area looking for donkeys as companions and as an economical way of keeping their grass short, Peter has a good supply of homes for the donkeys. Many others have retired to this beautiful part of the coast and left families behind in their native countries, and would like to offer a good home to a dog and a cat.

We both realized that with a climate like southern Portugal's it would be so easy for them to grow a whole medicine cupboard with the right help. The most common physical problems I see in abandoned dogs and cats abroad are conditions such as mange, ticks and fleas, and sarcoptic mange in neglected donkeys, and I make up a very useful remedy to help them. Aloe vera can help enormously, and garlic can keep sand flies at bay, immediately reducing the incidence of leishmaniasis, a parasitic disease which is already rife on the Mediterranean coast.

I was very excited at the prospect of being able to pass on my skills and leave a lasting legacy with Peter. I began to pack.

The preparation work involved for a trip abroad is enormous, and the night before I leave for the airport I spend hours in the apothecary making up a basic topical application of fresh aloe vera. With hundreds of plants to choose from scattered around the house, I pick several large, ripe, juicy leaves and liquidize them in the blender as a thick base for the various ingredients I will need when I'm at the rescue centres. The aloe vera is so fresh that it has to be kept in the fridge until the minute I'm on the way to the airport. In the early hours of the morning, on the way to the airport, I have been known to turn the car round and go back for the chilling bottles of aloe vera; these days I have a huge sticker on the fridge to remind me not to forget them.

The aloe vera plant is one of the four emblems on the coat of arms of the Royal College of Veterinary Surgeons, which shows just how much the RCVS respects the versatility of this plant as well as the medicinal properties of all plant life. One vet student in his final year at veterinary college, who brought his dog to me for a consultation, told me that one of his lecturers, a veterinary surgeon at London College, regularly uses aloe vera and happily recommends it to his students.

Ideally I like to use dark glass bottles for my potions and I have to wrap them carefully so they don't break in my suitcase. I use glass to avoid the possibility of the endocrine disruptor bisphenol A (BPA), which is present in some of the cheaper plastic bottles, leaching into my lovely organic mixtures.

When I arrived at the donkey sanctuary I immediately recognized that this was a place run by people who really understood and respected animals. It was fairly well hidden and well off the beaten track, with no signage outside. Peter is only too well aware that there are very few animal sanctuaries to accommodate the ever-increasing numbers of stray animals dumped on doorsteps, as can happen with some rescue centres. He told me how even though it is a well-kept secret, they still find plastic bags full of kittens outside. He had found a donkey tethered to the door one morning, and a family of dogs which had been thrown over the fence on another. I'm afraid that dumping animals at rescue centres in the expectation that the workers there will care for them happens all too often.

I loved the fact that it was all so open. The dogs and cats were separated, with the cattery on one side, but the dogs were free to run together in an open-plan, well-fenced set of pounds. Those with particular behaviour issues were kept separately or partnered with suitable companions, but around 15 dogs were sitting completely free on the veranda. Dogs will always sort out their place in the pack, although the carers observe them all the time. It was clear everyone knew the psychology of each dog and had split the pack accordingly.

I unpacked my bags of oils and set straight to work in Peter's kitchen. This was like Christmas for Peter! Bottle after bottle of the extraordinary aloe vera base lotion, with its almost psychedelic green colour, was now covering his kitchen table. I munched on some dried rose hips as I worked, and offered some to Peter, who was surprised at how much he liked the flavour. I told him that I never feed an animal berries, hips or herbs that I would not eat myself, and he heartily agreed. He couldn't wait to get stuck in with mixing in the local plants, and immediately dispatched one of the younger helpers to go and get some garlic. She came back with a string of the biggest bulbs of garlic I had ever seen. The smell was overpowering. This was local, gorgeous garlic and I was sure the aroma alone would keep the flies away.

Many of the dogs, cats and donkeys there were suffering from flea, mange, sarcoptic mange and tick issues, so I set about making up a treatment. I asked for a huge pot for the aloe vera, and for one of the helpers to grind the garlic in a huge pestle and mortar. I had a little production line set up there, and Peter was more than happy to let me delegate. He knew that I was here to work and he let me get on with it. He trusted me implicitly after the long conversation we had had on the phone. I had sent him a long email listing what I was bringing so that he could be sure that they wouldn't contra-indicate in the case of an animal already on medication. Peter's vet knew of my visit and was more than happy for me to share my expertise in healing and zoopharmacognosy.

Using Peter's blender, I blitzed the beaten garlic with water, and mixed up the citronella, neem and yarrow that I had brought from the UK with the fresh aloe vera concentrate that I had made at my apothecary. Carrying the mixture out to the donkeys in huge vats, we sponged down their flanks and around the back of their legs, taking care not to get the mixture anywhere near their eyes or genitals. I could see the donkeys' relief immediately as the flies flew off. They had been swarming with them in the 100-degree heat.

After we sponged them with the garlic lotion, the donkeys were going mad for the rose hips I was offering them by hand. I always make sure that animals can help themselves to herbs, never putting herbs in their water trough or trying to influence animals' choice in any way. These donkeys were clearly selecting the highly nutritious rose hips, a natural plant remedy in the wild. Varieties of wild roses grow all over the world and they all have high vitamin C content. Before these donkeys were rescued, they had very little vegetation to forage so were depleted of the vital nutrients needed to sustain them.

They also loved the seaweed, which contains many minerals and electrolytes to balance fluid retention – vital in hot weather. I placed a couple of buckets of fresh water in their corral, and added a couple of handfuls of dried seaweed hand-harvested from the French Atlantic so they could take what they needed in their own time. I stood back to watch as each one muscled in on the action and slurped the cool seaweed drink.

Most of the donkeys were over 20 years old and suffered from musculoskeletal problems, stiff joints and very brittle hooves, and I noticed that they were selecting devil's claw, a natural anti-inflammatory which soothes pain. Devil's claw also helps with the secretion of mucosa in the lining of the gut to aid digestion, something that older animals often need help with.

We then set off towards the dogs basking on the veranda. There were a number of different issues here, some which I could hardly believe. Sam, for example, a beautiful golden Labrador cross, had been deliberately set alight in his last home and had lost his fur. In that heat, he was getting sunburnt. The cooling lotion of aloe vera with yarrow and peppermint was an immediate relief. The look on his face said, 'Thank you.' Peter told me that Sam was still in shock from the episode with his previous owner and had been mute since arriving at the sanctuary. I did a full healing on him and he lapped it up.

As Sam slept in the shade after his healing, we sponged the mange and tick treatment onto the other dogs, again taking care to avoid the genitals and eyes. Flies and other foreign bodies can cause all sorts of problems with the eyes, such as conjunctivitis, so I made up a separate remedy for these infections. With any eye problem, it's vital to see the vet straight away, but this was an emergency first-aid situation as we didn't have access to one immediately. I made an eyebath out of mineral water and a few drops of sandalwood. It's a very gentle remedy, but I made sure that I only used it *around* the eye rather than directly on it. If I have to do anything with the eye itself, such as remove a foreign body, I always use a sterile saline solution and add some freshly prepared rose-petal water, using a sterile dropper pipette for the eye rinse. Interestingly enough, some animals self-select cornflower water, which helps with eye problems like cataracts.

I take my tins of sardines wherever I go, and as I was introduced to some of the dogs I offered some to each of them by hand. In that kind of heat, it's unrealistic to put sardines out in the feeding bowls because of the flies, and for once I understood that these animals have to be fed a dried-food diet because of the sheer number of dogs there. But with dried food come the skin problems, and some of the dogs were suffering from itchy, flaky skin. As I offered my macerated oils to them, those with itchy skin went mad for the calendula, which is known for its anti-inflammatory properties and its beneficial effect on the skin.

We left the dogs to snooze and headed into a barn to see Susie, a very old donkey, well into her thirties. Peter was obviously very fond of her. I could see that she was unable to get up, and agreed with Peter that she might well be dying. She had been lying down for 12 hours by that time, and although she was trying to rock her body back onto her feet, she just didn't have the strength any more. Peter was worried that she would get festering sores if we couldn't get her up, which would attract flies. If these were to be her last days, he wanted her to be comfortable.

I asked him to get the biggest bath towels he had, to use as hoists, and we carefully placed bales of straw on either side to keep Susie upright and to prevent her falling heavily onto her major organs. We also had to be careful that she didn't fall on us as we prepared to get her standing again. A few moments later Peter came back with two big bath towels and I arranged for three people to be on either side of Susie as we eased them underneath her. It was vital that we got her up on her front legs first, and we had to be very coordinated, with the right balance of people on each side.

She was so weak, bless her, and was swaying back and forth. She must have had such a strong will to get to her thirties in Portugal, where life is really hard on donkeys. With each of us holding a corner of a bath towel, we hoisted her up and held her there for about half an hour. She closed her eyes and allowed us to hold her, breathing freely again for the first time in hours. Gradually we took the front towel away, and spent a further half-hour supporting her back end. Finally we took the second towel away and, to everyone's amazement, she stayed up.

I was under no illusions. This was an old girl on her last legs, and I wasn't surprised to hear from Peter that by the time I was home again in England, she had passed over. The vet had been coming to see another animal there and Peter had asked him to euthanize her. It had been an enormous effort for her to get up, and without the ability to move and breathe freely her quality of life was badly impaired, but I was so pleased to have been able to spend those last hours with her, and to share in such a wonderfully cooperative loving moment with her friends at the sanctuary.

We at the Sanctuary are very glad to be working with the Healing Animals Organisation and we believe that Elizabeth and her organization have great symmetry with our charity. We run our farm in a slightly 'holistic' manner which, unlike many other charities, allows the majority of our animals to run free in large enclosures. We are the oldest animal charity in the Algarve, and we believe that we have achieved this by allowing our development to be flexible and are always open to new ideas. We welcomed Elizabeth and her ideas with open minds, and we have to say we were impressed. Although we have our own fully stocked pharmacy, operating theatre and vets' assistants, we recognize that animal pharmaceuticals can only provide some of the answers to the problems we face. Indeed, many of our animals have not just faced physical cruelty but mental also, which takes much longer to heal.

Elizabeth arrived like a breath of fresh air and brought us not only donations, which of course are desperately needed, but also rose hips, which our donkeys love, bags of devil's claw and other natural products. Our dogs also responded very positively to the natural oils and other products. We look forward to her return. We are also looking forward to receiving students of hers over the next year to work with us over here. This collaboration between our two

*organizations is one that we wish to continue and we look forward to
seeing our relationship develop further in the near future.*

PETER

Life Is for Living

> *All animals – except man – know that the principal
> business of life is to enjoy it.*
> SAMUEL BUTLER

Animals are much more 'in the moment' than most of their
human companions, and we can learn a great deal from them
about how to deal with illness. Despite the comfortable lives
they lead compared to their ancestors in the wild, their DNA
has preserved their instinct and 'survival of the fittest' is still
the whip that drives them through life, no matter how they're
feeling. As a result it is extremely difficult to tell when a bird
is ill, because its instinct programmes it to avoid any show
of vulnerability. Similarly, a dog or cat suffering from cancer
in the wild would put up with the pain and just get on with
life.

Samba, the Working Dog

Humans have a totally different relationship with illness than
animals have, and sometimes I have to teach this to a client in
order for their pet to regain his normal lifestyle again. Samba, a
beautiful ten-year-old spaniel cross, worked as a fully trained
companion for the deaf until she developed throat cancer.
Her owner, Lisa, and Jenny, one of my graduate healers,
brought her to me to complement the conventional treatment

and palliative care Samba was getting from her vet. I told Lisa that although both Jenny and I would do our best, the prognosis was not good. The cancer was already beginning to spread to the jaw and I knew that most vets won't touch the mandible joint. This was clearly terminal.

I see many patients – both human and animal – who are suffering from cancer and who come to me to raise their quality of life while they can. Neither they nor I have any expectation of a cure, but for many of them the healing can be life changing. As I settled Samba in my clinic, Lisa told me that the dog had been retired from working with the deaf since the onset of her illness. I felt terribly strongly that this was not what Samba would have chosen. She may have had cancer, but she still had a job to do. Lisa, naturally, had wrapped her in cotton wool as soon as they had been given the diagnosis, and was clearly devastated, but Samba simply wanted to get back to her life. Lisa seemed surprised at my suggesting this, but after some initial anxiety agreed to let Samba go back to work and help out at some local demonstrations.

With Samba fulfilled in her work again, it was Lisa who was no longer filled with pain and sadness. Her change in mood seemed to contribute to the healings that she was getting from myself and Jenny. When Lisa rang a few months later to say that the vet's x-ray showed that the tumour in Samba's jaw had partially disappeared, I wasn't surprised.

Our animals are so like us in many respects and have many of the same kinds of illnesses and emotional problems, but it's important not to foist too many human attributes onto our animals. A little anthropomorphism can help us understand what we have in common with our pets; recognizing that a rescued animal is going to be confused and grieving is going to help as he settles into his new life, but treating him like a depressive for months on end won't. Dogs, like children, want to live in the now, and we can learn a great deal from them.

PART FOUR
Death Is Not the End

I often build up a relationship with a client over several years, and the animals can become so intimate with me that I feel like part of the family. When the phone rings to tell me that an animal has passed over, I feel that great loss, too. I reflect back on our time together and feel so proud to have known that beautiful animal and to be helping his soul on to the next life. For me, it is an honour to be a part of the cycle of life.

I like to light a candle, say a prayer and visualize the soul energy passing over peacefully on its journey. Of course the owner will be feeling bereaved and often will be in shock, harbouring a feeling of not wanting to let go. This is all part of the grieving process, and supporting people through distant healing and bereavement counselling can help them come to terms with their loss. At whatever stage I am needed, I am there for my clients and for the whole family.

Lucy and Ralph

When it is the human owner who is ill and the pet that is the bereaved, I am also there. When I first met Lucy and her gorgeous lurcher cross, Ralph, he was very anxious and wouldn't leave her side. He sat right next to her rather than sniff around as most dogs do when they come to my clinic. She smiled down at him and explained that he was her bodyguard, that when they were out on a walk, he never bounded off but stayed right next to her.

She explained that she was very ill, and she believed that Ralph knew this. She had been born with an extremely rare heart condition and knew that she could die at any time. As is often the case with people who grow up understanding the fragility of life, Lucy was a beautiful soul, a young woman who even though she was only in her early twenties, had an air of wisdom and grace around her that is deeply unusual.

As we went through Ralph's history, Lucy told me that he had always suffered from a very delicate stomach. The rescue centre had found him dumped at the end of their driveway at three weeks old, five weeks before a healthy weaning should take place, so they had very little history. The manager told Lucy that Ralph had been very quiet and subdued until she had arrived, and she remembered how he had walked towards the edge of his pound to greet her.

I noticed the concerned look in his eyes. He was agitated, pacing around the room, settling right next to Lucy for a moment before pacing again. I felt that Ralph was picking up on her increasing fragility and understood how weak she was. As I began the attunement, he began to settle down, and I felt the stress and grief pouring out of him. It felt as if his heart was already breaking.

Lucy told me that she had been going back and forth to hospital recently, and Ralph had become increasingly anxious.

She seemed to find the guided meditation very peaceful and relaxing, but every breath she took was a considerable strain on her body. As she relaxed more deeply, so did Ralph, his eyes softening and for a brief moment, closing. He knew that Lucy was in safe hands.

After the healing session, Lucy was intrigued by Ralph's interest in my tool box filled with macerated oils and floral waters. I had just macerated some rose hips and the aroma was so delicious that as I poured a little of this rich jewel in the crown of oils onto a ceramic plate, Ralph soon polished it off, looking at me for more. He sniffed at the rose-water bottle as I tipped a little on another saucer and inhaled the smells of the delicate rose petals deeply, his eyes glowing and his coat shining. I explained to Lucy how each part of the rose plant plays a different but vital role to create balance in the body. The rose hips are robust and packed full of vitamins and antioxidants to maintain a healthy immune system when stressed, while the rose water, delicate yet soft, works very deeply on the emotions of the heart that so easily get bruised. Roses have a wonderful capacity to lift our spirits and are completely intoxicating. There is nothing like smelling a rose in full bloom, with so many aromas in one head.

I felt she had such a wonderful passion for animals and plants, and asked her what she wanted to do with the rest of her life. She loved the idea of working with complementary therapies for animals, especially anything to do with the vibrational aspect of plant remedies. She had watched Ralph making a beeline for most parts of the rose plant and ignoring other oils like violet leaf, neroli and calendula macerated oil, and a light bulb had gone on in her head. She needed something to get her teeth into while she was in hospital so regularly and unable to work, and I was thrilled when she rang me some weeks later to tell me that she had enrolled in a course which incorporated Bach flower remedies at the University of Southampton. Ralph had opened a door for her and given her something to put her special energy into.

A few months later, Lucy's mother, Suzi, called to tell me that she had gone. Ralph was now staying with Lucy's husband, who was in pieces after the loss of his beautiful young wife. I told her that if there was anything I could do for anyone in the family, I was available.

It was almost a year later when Suzi rang to tell me that Ralph really wasn't doing well. She told me that Lucy had said how much she and Ralph had enjoyed my healing sessions, and wondered whether I could come to the house to see if I could help him again. I could hear the grief in Suzi's voice but she couldn't ask for help for herself or for her husband Charlie. They were both in their early fifties and the pain that they were going through in losing their beautiful daughter was heart-breaking.

A few weeks after Lucy's death, Ralph moved out of his family home and in with Suzi and Charlie. He was pining terribly and they all hoped that Lily, Suzi and Charlie's golden Labrador, might be able to cheer him up. And, bless her, she tried. She would bring him her toys and offer to play by throwing her teddy around, nudge him with her nose, or just curl up next to him, but Ralph wouldn't rise out of his gloom. He didn't growl at her; he simply retreated. Worst of all, he was refusing to eat.

When I got to the house, Suzi was out; apparently she had forgotten that I was coming. Charlie ushered me into a room with Lily and Ralph, muttered something about having something to do, and left me with the two dogs.

I settled down on the floor and was greeted by Lily first. She came over and gave me a huge lick and rolled over, asking for her belly to be rubbed. She looked over her shoulder at Ralph who was quietly watching from a distance. As I began to tune in to Ralph, I could feel his overwhelming grief, but he refused to accept my healing. Instead, Lily remained by my side and placed her head into my outstretched hands, drew in a deep breath, sank deeper into the carpet and relished this time for herself. I could sense that Charlie and Suzi were finding it very hard to get through this difficult time, and Lily had been busy trying to comfort them all.

As the stillness fell and Lily relaxed right down, something changed in the room. Suddenly Ralph pricked up his ears, his eyes shining as he looked past me. Lucy's energy was very clearly in the room. It was so strong. It was if she was there with us. It was a deep honour to be a part of such a special moment; the love in that room was not something that you come across very often. Lucy had taken total responsibility for herself with such bravery and such grace. She was an enlightened soul whose love for her dog was unconditional.

Suzi rang the next day to apologize for not having been there, and told me that Ralph was a changed dog. He had gone out for a walk with Lily and Charlie that morning, something he hadn't done since Lucy's death, and was playing with Lily as if he was a puppy. And he was eating again.

Ralph was lucky; even though Suzi and Charlie were not personally interested in healing, they were prepared to support Lucy's philosophy even after her death and Ralph is now a beautifully balanced and happy dog in his new home.

I have witnessed the most fabulous strength among my clients – animal and human – at times of bereavement, and I would like to pay tribute to them all in this book. Illness is a harsh teacher but there is a great sense of achievement when we have pulled through a terrible illness, either ourselves or when healing our loved ones. We could learn a thing or two from the way that our pets handle life and death.

> *Elizabeth is exceptionally kind and gifted when healing animals – and humans. Just one example of this was Ralph, a beautiful rescue lurcher cross who belonged to my daughter Lucy. Lucy sadly died just over three years ago, and Ralph came to live with us. He was pining terribly, but thanks to Liz's healing he has recovered well and has a new start in life. All of us have benefited from this. Long may her work continue.*
> SUZI

Brucie and Me

My healing career began when I was convinced that I could help Wow to recover from his horrific accident. But perhaps my real life's work began when I had to make the ultimate decision about my beautiful boxer, Bruce. I tell my students that it is with empathy rather than sympathy that we offer healing to animals and their owners, and my pain and my ability to let Bruce die were my greatest lesson.

Bruce was my boy. He was a typical boxer, full of love and energy, and we adored each other. So when he came back from a routine trip to the vet to have some teeth out, I was shattered to find him paralysed from the waist down. The vet had taken out more teeth than expected from our initial consultation, and I believe that it was the strength of the anaesthetic used that had paralysed Bruce. He seemed to have lost everything that he had been: that pride, that vitality and bouncy boxer energy were all gone. Bruce was only eight years old. Only the previous week he had been in perfect health and now, suddenly, I did not know what life had in store for him. I knew that I was pouring my energy into these thoughts rather than thinking about what Bruce needed me to do, but for a short while at least, I sobbed until I thought my heart would break.

Finally, I banished the negative thoughts from my mind, dusted myself down and focused on what to do for him. This was not about me, but about my unconditional love for Bruce. I had taught this for years by then to my clients and my students, and this now was my own biggest challenge.

I settled down to heal him. I began working on his adrenals to ground his energies, and I held back the tears as Bruce shuffled his front legs around so I could heal his stomach. I willed myself to send waves of love as I relieved the pressure of his abdomen weighing heavily on his organs. He sighed and lay flat out, his soft, big brown eyes watching my every move, soulful and approving. I willed his back legs to work, but muscle atrophy was already setting in on the hind limbs, and they lay lifeless. He only had movement from his strong front limbs, and he drank up the healing at the shoulders, which were taking the bulk of the strain of pulling himself around.

This was something that I couldn't do alone, so I called in the troops: my network of healers, students and friends, who were only too pleased to help. Bruce loved all the attention and healing as equine osteopath Elizabeth Oakenfold joined Jacquie Wilton, training manager of The National Federation of Spiritual Healers, and my students in a wonderful healing meditation. While we held our vigil for Bruce in Sussex, his name was placed on healing lists from Cornwall to the US as my emails spread across the globe.

I was tremendously strengthened by this caring, supportive network, physically as well as mentally. And I needed it: when Bruce needed to relieve himself, I had to lift him outside. We knew each other well after eight years together. He only needed to give me a look and I would place a sheepskin wrap under his abdomen and raise his back legs up so he could walk with his front legs. But at more than seven stone, he was a big boy; it was times like this I wished he was the size of Alf and I could have carried him in my arms.

I put on a brave face and kept smiling at him as we made the best of the time we had left. I was determined to give him whatever he needed, including my positive energy. I could feel his frustration. His body was functioning well from the front end; when an insect landed on his nose, he was quick to swipe it with his front paw. But it was his back end that wasn't working, and this had been his engine, his powerhouse. He was already expending a great deal of energy and putting a strain on his front limbs and paws, so I bought what I could to support him, including fitted boots which looked like a pair of flat boxing gloves to help protect his front pads. That little boxer loved them and raised one paw at a time to let me put them on. He loved my massages, and the daily exercise programme I had worked out to stimulate his blood supply and circulation and to keep the muscles functioning.

After three weeks Bruce started to lose control of his bladder. He was eating and drinking well, breathing normally and otherwise completely alert, but Dominic (my vet) and I were by now having regular discussions. I asked him to come for a home visit to check that Bruce was OK, and he reassured me that Bruce was very comfortable and didn't need any medication. He was impressed with the daily routine, even with the disposable nappies – which, surprisingly, did a very good job. He understood the agonizing decisions that lay ahead of me and Brian, and placed his hand on my arm and told me that he was there for us any time. I tucked Bruce up and went to my bedroom where I could cry my heart out without him seeing me. I knew that he would have been worried for me.

I searched my soul for the reason why I couldn't heal my own dog. The healings were making no difference to his back legs at all. I knew that it was working on him – and me – on other levels, but after all the animals I had healed over the years, I couldn't bear the fact that I couldn't save my own beloved dog. I reminded myself that so much of healing has to do with letting go, making the energy become lighter and lighter until the challenges facing both owner and pet become effortless, even if these challenges are death and bereavement.

I pulled myself together and started to make plans. I asked my mum and sister Susi if Alf could stay with them for a holiday, knowing that he would be well looked after while Brian and I could spend Bruce's last days with him. Alf loved going to stay with them; my sister would take him for regular walks on his favourite beach and my mum had stocked up on all his favourite food.

I shut up the clinic and postponed my patients' appointments so that I could devote all my energy to Bruce. I even bought a pram so that he could continue his 'walks' in the countryside with me, all seven stone of boxer dog. He loved to be out and about with me, and if it looked ridiculous, we didn't care. For the next five days I spent every moment of the day and night with my beautiful boy. Time stood still, every single moment was precious and fun. Even as I was preparing to teach the diploma in animal healing, counting out the student module papers in piles on the living room floor, Bruce was by my side, nosing at everything that was going on around him. I played healing music and lit candles and we relished this time together.

A few days later I noticed that Bruce had refused his breakfast and had failed to give me his usual nod to go outside. He was lying listlessly in his bed, looking at me with his deep brown eyes. Tears welled up in my eyes as he tapped his front paw on the duvet to bring me to him and he placed his paw on my hand. I couldn't hold back the tears any longer and hugged him tightly, sobbing quietly into his soft fur. We both knew that it was time.

I had asked Dominic to euthanize him at home, and had prepared the space, with candles around his comfy duvet on the floor. Bruce lay there, calm and peaceful as I began one final healing, wave after wave of pure, unconditional love floating between us until finally, very gently, I could feel him begin to let go. By the time that Brian showed Dominic in to see us, I could tell that Brucie was already leaving us. As Dominic gave him the injection, we all knew that it was almost unnecessary.

I am so grateful to Bruce for being in my life and the bond we shared. I never gave it a second thought about the round-the-clock care that was needed towards the end of his life. As a treasured member of my family he deserved nothing but the best, however hard it was to deal with emotionally and physically. I take full responsibility as a pet guardian to help all my animals through illness to old age, including the financial implications and time. When anybody makes a commitment to give a pet a home, however long or short that time is we owe it to every animal to give it the best quality of life. I find it very sad when some people refuse to take notice of their animal's needs.

When I look at Alf now, at 14 he still looks like a young pup. However, he has changed and over time he has slowed down with age, a little stiff in his hind legs, leisurely taking his time on a walk and sleeping most of the day. Like us he feels the cold in the winter months and gingerly steps outside and visibly shakes until he warms up. I deliberately do not clip him between November and March as I want to keep him well insulated with his wiry coat. I just cannot imagine life without him, he has been such a trusted and loyal friend who has been with me through thick and thin, and yet I realize that death and dying are a natural part of life for us and for animals, and when that time comes I will let Alf go gracefully and in a dignified manner.

Euthanasia is the humane option for terminally ill animals, or for those with a poor quality of life that can't be improved through veterinary assistance. I encourage my clients to consider allowing their animals to pass away peacefully at home if possible, and there are many vets who agree to do this, knowing how much more comforting and comfortable it is for all concerned. If euthanasia has to be carried out at the veterinary practice, it is possible to ask for an appointment at the end of the day when it is quieter, and when the owners can have the time to say a proper goodbye.

Polly and Maxwell

I performed a healing on my friend Polly's beautiful 14-year-old cross-breed, Maxwell, as he passed away in a quiet corner of her vet's surgery. He was an old wolf of a dog, the prime example of a cross-breed: strong and lean throughout his life with not a day of illness until his 13th year. Arthritis had recently begun to weaken his back legs, but he had been bright and alert until the day he died, even popping into his local pet shop for a sniff of a pig's ear on his way to the vet.

Polly had called me because Maxwell had been behaving oddly during the night, panting heavily and insisting on sitting outside the house, despite the ice on the ground, and gazing out across his territory. She had cuddled him for most of the night, the two of them wrapped in an old fake-fur coat, listening to the sounds of the night together, in spite of the cold.

She had rung the vet first thing in the morning to see if his medication should be changed, and I met her at the vet's to see if I could help. Maxwell wagged his tail and came to welcome me as he had always done, despite obvious discomfort. As the vet talked to Polly I put my hands close to his body and he settled into a healing with a sigh, lying still and calm while the vet conducted her examination. She found no obvious reason for his panting, and referred him for a scan. He walked away with her, relaxed and calm, without a backward glance despite his long-held fear of vets.

When the vet called to say that he was in heart failure and that she recommended putting him down immediately, we were all in a state of shock, but rushed back to the surgery where he had been sedated and kept comfortable in a quiet corner. Polly and her husband joined me in a final healing as the vet gave Maxwell the injection, and we watched him gently slip away, giving thanks for who he was, the life he'd led, for everything that they had given each other in this life. The vet, who knows my work well, watched quietly before leaving Polly and her husband with Maxwell for as long as they needed. I wasn't surprised to hear that she had sent a bereavement card to them the following week.

Polly had always wanted to allow Maxwell to pass away at home, but when the time came they did what was best for him, not them. They brought his body home and buried him in the garden he'd loved so much, with a small ceremony and a beautiful grave which is already scampered over by Polly's rescue pups, one of whom has something about her which looks remarkably like old Maxwell.

Amy and Bella

I have conducted many ceremonies at the homes of my clients whose pets have passed over – on one occasion I've even helped to dig a grave!

An owner and I will spend time together planning the ceremony, just as you would for a person's funeral, and this can include poetry, songs and hymns. Many owners feel that a funeral is not appropriate for an animal, despite how broken-hearted they feel. I believe that all momentous occasions should be well marked; a ceremony can be a tremendously cathartic experience, and can allow a pet owner to move on to a new phase in his or her life.

Amy, a 78-year-old artist whose work had been prolific until her husband died, found that she was able to paint again after the funeral of her 17-year-old cat, Bella. Bella had been refusing to eat and had become very thin in her old age, and it was clear that it was her time to go. But Amy had had Bella since she was a kitten and couldn't bear the thought of life without her. Still mourning for her husband, who had died the year before, she was comforted by Bella's companionship and friendship. Bella, equally devoted to Amy, was holding on. Neither of them was able to let the other go.

Amy invited me to her house and, over the next four months, I conducted many healings on Bella. Amy enjoyed having the opportunity to chat. I noticed her arthritic hands and wondered whether this had anything to do with her artist's block. I offered to do some healing on her, too, and she happily accepted. Amy loved to see Bella so relaxed during the healings and lick delicately at the tinned fish as she regained her appetite. These healing sessions were incredibly important in allowing allow Amy to think about Bella's best interests, to deal with her fear of the unknown and to enable her to talk openly with her trusted vet and seek his advice every step of the way.

When Bella started to lose interest in food again, Amy asked me if I would come and do one final healing. They both knew that it was time. We sat down in Amy's light, airy lounge, sunlight flooding through the window. I began to attune. Bella seemed tired and ready to pass over, but anxious about Amy. She kept opening her eyes to check on her before settling down again.

As they both relaxed deeply, Amy's tears finally came. I gave her some tissues and she cried like a child. When her sobs had finally subsided, she sighed and told me that Bella's favourite place in the garden was the magnolia tree, and we both knew that this was where she would like her ashes to be scattered. She and Bella looked at each other with a new understanding.

After the healing, I suggested that she talk to the vet and ask him to visit Bella in the comfort of her own home, something Amy didn't know was possible. Allowing Bella to die in her arms made all the difference to Amy, and I could feel the gentle release beginning to take place between the two of them. I suggested she organize a pet funeral for Bella, a celebration of her life which I felt would be an enormously important part of letting her go. It would also give Amy something creative to focus on over the next week.

Bella's funeral was beautifully simple and peaceful. I asked Amy if I could read the prayer of Francis of Assisi, the patron saint of animals, and Amy's tears were flowing freely now. She had let go of the fear of losing her best friend and the painful restrictions in her cramped, controlled body were beginning to ease as she let her grief melt. Her friends and family joined in a celebration of Bella's life, putting her right at the heart of the past 17 years of Amy's fascinating life as an artist, wife and mother, her companion and guide.

As Bella's ashes were buried under the magnolia tree on that gorgeous autumn afternoon, we all looked out over the Sussex countryside and remembered all the pets and people who had guided us through our own journeys, and thanked Amy and Bella for giving us that moment of peace and reflection.

A few weeks later Amy rang to ask for another healing and told me that she had been painting again. Her creative block had shifted. Even her arthritic hands had loosened up. She accepts that she is alone now; at 78, she knows that she can't have another cat in her life to replace her Bella. But she has her art again, and the memory of a beautiful death to help the long bereavement process.

Carrington

Most animals – like humans – do not easily accept their own mortality, so it was another of my great lessons when Carrington, an elderly bay, taught me what it is to know when it's time to go.

This beautiful old horse had been taken in by Pip, who had heard that he needed a retirement home after riding the hunt for years. When I first met him, he had settled into Pip's herd after a tricky start, thanks to her gorgeous chestnut mare, Holly. At 17.2 hands, Holly is built like a brick house and takes no prisoners. When Carrington started kicking the other smaller horses around, it was Holly who put him right. It was as if she said, 'Look, mate, if you want to be with me, you need to know how it works around here.' She was the undisputed boss and he loved her.

Pip looked after them all very well; they had plenty of turn-out and a warm, cosy stable at night. But there was something about Carrington that I had not seen before.

I have met aggressive horses before, but this was different. Pip had called me in because Carrington seemed to keep everyone – even Holly – at a distance. He wouldn't let any vets or therapists near him, and I approached him very carefully, grounding myself, breathing in love and breathing out love.

He looked at me as if to say, 'OK, what's your game?' As I began to attune and place my hands near his stomach and neck, checking for hot and cool points, I could feel heat where there was inflammation, cold spots where there was a blockage in his energy, and huge pulsations in my palms as the energy flowed through.

He began to relax right down, resting his back leg and sighing. Pip couldn't believe that Carrington was letting me work on his stifles and hocks at the back of his body. Horses show their disdain by turning a rear end to warn that they can kick good and hard if they need to, and Pip had never seen Carrington let anyone near him before. I scanned his skeletal frame and felt the arthritis in his joints, and the many places on his body where he had been abused. He was showing me where he had been hit and whipped, and where he had hardened in a bid for self-preservation. But it was more than pain; what I was picking up felt like a huge weight that he was carrying in his tired old body.

Animals often show us how natural our own responses can be; we also harden to protect ourselves. We place a coat of armour around ourselves, often from an early age, and it's a completely natural response. After I had spent some time healing him, though, he seemed to open up to me. It felt like blowing up a balloon and seeing its shape come into being. His coat was already beginning to shine as he leaned in closer to me, encouraging me to work more deeply.

When I am healing I am usually utterly focused, and so the chill that I suddenly felt seemed to come completely out of the blue. I felt that this horse did not want to be here any more. I was shocked. Every animal struggles for survival, but here was one who had simply given up. I asked Pip why he might feel so defeated, and she told me that his former owner had been a huntsman and driven Carrington into the ground. When his tired old body could no longer keep up with the others after years of service, the huntsman had wanted to feed his carcass to the hounds, as is the tradition in some hunting societies.

I could tell that Carrington felt it really hard to forgive. He had lost faith in humans; that man had broken Carrington's spirit. I breathed in love and breathed out love and he took as much healing as he could. He suddenly began to empty his bowels, to Pip's utter amazement. She told me that he had had stomach problems until now and been unable to pass stools easily, but here he was really letting go. I had helped him to help himself, to ground himself, to protect himself and to clear out what he needed to in order to move on. He nuzzled me and I hugged him.

As I was about to leave, I noticed that Pip had broken her ankle and asked her if she was getting any physio. I knew she worked in the fractures department of a hospital but that she was one of those people who put themselves at the bottom of their own list of priorities. I suggested that she take responsibility for her own health, not just for her sake, but for her animals' and her family, and offered her a healing. She laughed and quickly dismissed it. She's a typical no-nonsense horsey woman and the idea of being healed was far too out of her comfort zone, despite having just seen the effects on her old horse. Finally, I insisted, telling her that I had found it such an honour healing Carrington that I wanted to thank her in the best way I knew.

A few weeks later she came to the clinic for her appointment, and tearfully told me that Carrington had passed over the week before. He had done very well after the healing, his coat glistening and his attention much sharper than she had seen before, but he was just too worn out to go on.

I took her upstairs to my healing room. I had spent half an hour meditating before she'd arrived and had blessed the room, lit the candles and put on some gentle music. As Pip lay down on the couch, she floated off almost immediately and the room filled with a beautiful light energy. Carrington was there for a very brief but incredible moment. It's not something that I experience often, and I have to say that for a second I struggled to keep my composure. I have some private moments to shed my tears, but there are times when I want to cry my eyes out from the sheer potency of the moment. This was one, but I didn't want Carrington to feel that he had put too much of a burden on me, so I steeled myself and breathed the love in and out until I could bring Pip back into the room. I gave her some water which I had already blessed to ground her energies, and we went downstairs.

We were in the kitchen afterwards chatting about the healing over a cup of tea when very quietly she told me about a strange feeling she had had. She said, 'Carrington came, didn't he?' I nodded and she cried again. I put my arms around her and this time we cried together; the healing was over and we were celebrating the life of a beautiful soul.

Death is not the end. It's the legacy of a beautiful friendship and the start of a new phase in our own development. My Bruce taught me so much about pain and letting go, and he guides me every day as my clinic builds and the healings spread out across the world.

The natural world, with its lessons in birth, death and rebirth, has so much to teach us, and the animals who live so harmoniously within it have much to tell us about. I am surrounded by my teachers: my journey started with my connection with Wow, who at 21 years old still inspires me in my work every day. Betty and her little foal, Iris, and her step-brother Dancer light up my life with their instinct and intuition, while Alf, Lily and Morris teach me every day about the lightness of being. Then there is Mrs T, quietly yet reassuringly watching over me and showing me how I too can hone my observation skills and remain focused and grounded in this world. They are my healers and my guides. This book is for them.

> *What is man without the beasts? If all beasts were gone,*
> *man would die from a great loneliness of spirit.*
> Chief Seattle of the Duwamish, Suquamish and allied tribes

PART FIVE
What We Know Now

It's been a long journey to where I am now, and I am so humbled by what my patients, both human and animals, have taught me over these last ten years. I spend a good deal of time meditating on these life lessons and considering what I know now, and perhaps one of the most important is a reminder to spend a little more time with those closest to me.

My husband Brian and I live very different lives and spend so much of the time apart from each other; I'm usually travelling all over the country – and, increasingly, the world – and when I'm at home, I'm normally in the clinic or with my students, even over the weekends. Our interests are also very different, but one thing that we're both passionate about is wildlife conservation. One beautiful warm summer evening in early July, we managed to find a rare moment when we were both at home together. We had spent the past few weeks listening to the screeching noises of the female barn owl who had taken up residence in the box Brian had made and placed on the side of the barn where I do much of my teaching.

For the past four years, we had been waiting for this glorious sound to fill our garden. Owls are becoming increasingly rare in the UK now, mainly due to lack of food, habitat and an increase in precipitation. Barn owl feathers are not very waterproof and therefore they cannot hunt in the rain, and often die due to starvation. The increase in rainfall due to climate change has had a knock-on effect with dwindling numbers of young; most mothers will now only raise one or two youngsters per nest.

But finally we could hear the tell-tale sounds of babies in the nest. Like viper snakes hissing, these owlets were hungry for food; we reckoned they could only be about five weeks old and we were thrilled at the thought of sharing our home with this precious little family. Grabbing a couple of old comfy chairs and some blankets, we stole out into the dusky evening to settle ourselves down to watch the mother at work.

The sand school sits at the edge of our drive, looking over to the horses' paddock in one direction, the woods in another and out over the barn, normally so filled with the activity and energy of my students, and now so quiet and calm. I love the 'left brain' buzziness of some of the students, the accountants and doctors who find the work that we do such a leap of faith. The way that education has trained them to think is a joy for me to work with; I adore science and technology and love to find new ways, inspired by my students, to marry them with healing and more 'right brain' ways of seeing the world. I smiled at the thought of the hundreds of people who have walked out of those barn doors with a clarity of purpose and a commitment to spreading the work that I have taught them across the world.

Brian and I put our chairs in the middle of the sand school, the sand still warm from the summer sunshine, and settled in for a night of owl watching. With our barn owl finally having come to roost in our home, this was a wonderful opportunity to cuddle up together and enjoy each other.

As the night drew in, the stars began to twinkle over this magical world in which I had learnt so much in the ten years we had been here. I looked over at the horses that I had led into the paddock a little earlier, to Wow, my guide, my soul mate and my mentor over all this time and gave a little prayer of thanks for our wonderful relationship. He was busy showing Iris, now 16 months old and full of curiosity, the hedgerows full of delicious herbs and goodness, while Dancer and Betty lazily stretched their legs after a day in the cool stable. With the summers getting hotter, I find that they prefer to spend their evenings grazing in the paddock, and I watched as they began to form a loose huddle, Betty and Dancer shielding little Iris, and Wow at the back, the observation post for any prey as the night continued to advance.

Brian nudged me urgently and put his finger to his lips to silence me as he pointed to a badger shyly edging out towards us. We had planted some trees around the sand school when we moved in all those years ago, and we watched in awe as the badger snuffled for food among the roots. The tranquillity of the evening was allowing me to observe the natural, peaceful way of life of these animals that I so rarely give myself time to enjoy, and it felt such an honour now to be able to share it with my lovely man. We smiled at each other and said nothing. We knew what it had taken to get to this point for both of us, how much loneliness for him, and how much commitment it has taken and sheer hard work it has been for me to set up the clinic and keep on the road I had chosen. So many relationships collapse when one partner is driven to follow a path. So many egos get in the way of friendship and understanding, but in that smile, we both acknowledged what it had taken for both of us to get to this wonderful moment now. I took his hand and held it for a very long time.

Suddenly the barn owl was right above us, her white feathered undercarriage and huge wingspan taking our breath away as she swooped into the woods, the night perfectly camouflaging her buff-coloured upper body. Every 15 minutes, she would return to her nest, pausing just long enough to deliver mice, field voles and shrews to her brood. Prey is swallowed whole by the owlets and the bones and fur are regurgitated, and I chuckled as I remembered showing Reg Lanaway, our ornithologist friend, a regurgitated pellet that I had mistaken for owl faeces. He had noticed the remains of a vole skull within the pellet, and recorded this information to gain insights on owl eating habits.

Brian and I longed to see how many owlets she had in there. I knew if they were about five weeks old they would be covered in soft white down fluff and have lovely heart shaped faces. As the owlets mature, these specialised feathers create a disc around the face to trap and focus sound which is handy when you are hunting the smallest of prey in the dense undergrowth. We knew it would be wrong to disturb them now. Brian Walter, the local barn owl specialist and ringer, and Reg had also been eager for owls to come to our barn and we would work with them to ring their legs to record them when the time was right.

Our female barn owl was hunting while flying, not wasting a second of her time. We could see from the countless journeys to and fro that she clearly had more than one mouth to feed, but we just had to be patient for now. I timed her trips; at first, every 15 minutes she would religiously return to her brood but I noticed that she was taking longer and longer as the evening wore on. We could hear the babies hissing after 15 minutes, becoming more urgent with each gap. I marvelled at the way that animals are so in tune with time, that their natural body clock is more punctual than most humans' could ever be, but I worried that this might mean that the mother owl had got into trouble. Brian squeezed my hand and told me to relax. 'This is nature at its best, and you've just got to trust it', he reminded me.

I stilled myself, remembering the cost of not taking responsibility for our own anxieties. How many times had I seen my human clients' issues projected onto their animals? How often had I noticed the world spinning out of its natural rhythm because of human intervention? I breathed slowly, reminding myself of my place in the natural order of things.

Brian smiled at me gently, knowing what I was battling with. It's a gift to have someone in my life who knows me so well. I looked around at the beautiful evening, the horses now in a close huddle, enjoying the warmth and security of their family, and the badger continuing to snuffle his way through the trees, and remembered my previous life in sales at *The Daily Mail* and in the pharmaceutical industry. I sighed with relief at how far I'd come. Every day I am thankful for having been strong enough to have found my way out of that lifestyle, and to have learnt the skills to heal those who are still there so that I can support them enough to find their own balance. I know now that people don't have to give up on their lives to find peace, that it's about finding their own way. We're all so similar in so many ways, but there isn't one quick fix that suits everyone. The animals and people who have come through the doors of my clinic have taught me to lose any judgement I had, and to remember that there are many roads to finding the sense of peace that I had come to right here.

She was back! 30 minutes had passed and the moon was now high in the night sky. The hissing of the babies – we guessed, breath held, that there were three – was shrill and urgent now against the silence of the woods. Brian and I were on the edge of our seats as she finally swooped over our heads to her brood. I was still worried that she had to go outside her territory to find her prey and remembered how heart-broken I had been earlier that day when I had taken the dogs into the nearby meadow, once filled with gorgeous wild flowers, a paradise for mice and small mammals until the farmer had sprayed it with weed killer, reducing its beauty to an apocalyptic wasteland in just 24 hours. I understand the need for farmers to maximise their crops, but the effect on the wildlife is critical now. We all know the impact on climate change and the future of the planet, and however beautiful the night was, my heart ached.

I'm absolutely passionate about conservation, and with a bedrock of students spreading my work out across the country and the world, I am now able to take myself out of my clinic and into areas of the world where whole species are at risk. The stories are for another time (and another book), but being invited to work with elephants whose limbs have been blown off in the civil war in Sri Lanka was one of my most humbling moments of the last year.

At the turn of the nineteenth century, there were approximately 18,000 elephants in Sri Lanka, but these have dwindled now to around 3000. Elephants have been such a loyal companion to the Sinhalese and have been domesticated for over 4000 years, often employed to pull large tree trunks through the jungle to the saw mills for export. Although a handful of elephants are still involved in the logging trade, newer forms of technology have taken over. It is illegal now in Sri Lanka to kill elephants, but it wasn't so long ago that they were hunted for pleasure, captured and destroyed because they were deemed agricultural pests. As food and water has become scarcer, wild elephants have increasingly been forced on to cultivated land and into conflict with man. The highly competent Sri Lankan Department of Wildlife Conservation has stepped in and is adopting conservation measures, one of which is to create more national parks throughout the country to avoid disturbing the distribution of some of the original herds.

As I led the elephant victims of the civil war into the river to cool down, I healed them one by one, my eyes filling up at the thought of the loss of these beautiful, gentle giants to the world. So many gorgeous creatures are now at risk because of human selfishness. Climate change is Mother Nature's answer to our irresponsible curiosity and our desire for more, and it's the animals, the plants and the trees that have always lived so harmoniously with each other that are the first to suffer.

Although it does make me angry, I'm not one of those people who give up on humans, and I believe that if people became more aware of the impact their actions have on the natural world, they would think twice. I have just come back from the Sinai where I was working with The Makhad Trust, a dedicated charity helping Bedouin tribes and their camels as the effects of climate change ravage the indigenous desert plants and local crops. Astonishingly, there has been just one day of rainfall in the last year and local tribe leaders are very worried about the future for their camels. The only food available to some of those at Mount Sinai is the cardboard packaging discarded by local shopkeepers, which camels can digest, but which has no nutritional value. Even most of the local water is conserved for the lucrative holiday industry three hours away at the seaside resort of Sharm el-Sheikh. Meanwhile camels, which need 60 litres of water every two days to fuel their journeys into the middle of the desert, are unable to find enough. I believe that if the holiday makers knew this, they could force change or at least give some extra cash to help the situation. It's for this reason that I have already set up Camel Aid (see www.healinganimals.org for details). Again, it's a story for another time, but I am so grateful to be able to help these beasts of burden at such a crucial time.

From the dolphins in Portugal to the race horses in Dublin and the Olympic show jumpers that I am also working with in Ireland, the work that I am able to do to prove the benefit of healing is only part of my mission. And it really is a mission. By encouraging owners and trainers to understand how a more holistic way of being can help any animal get more out of life, whether it's in competition like the retrievers at Crufts I've been working with, or prized Aberdeen Angus show breeds for county agricultural shows, the message about our essential relationship with nature becomes part of their lives too. You take more care of the countryside when you see the natural medicine it provides for your beloved animals, just as you take more care of your animal when you understand what it has been going through for you.

I realise now that I am only just beginning to do my work, and it is with all that I have absorbed from my animal and human patients that I continue on this fabulously exciting path. The dogs which, after hundreds of years of evolving into man's best friend, have shown me what loyalty really means, and the cats, the original domestic rat catchers, still remind me of the peace that true independence can bring. But it's the horses that for me are truly grounding, perhaps because I will never forget the legacy of my beautiful Wow and the journey we have already travelled together. I watch him now, proudly standing back as the grandfather of the herd, as Betty, the matriarch, leads Dancer, now nine years old and finally a responsible big brother after an extended single, and rather indulged, childhood, and Iris, the curious little foal, towards the natural herbal remedies of the hedgerows. Wow bends his beautiful head and looks over at me and, just for a moment, we know everything we need to know.

PART SIX

Recipes

K9/Feline Fishcakes

1 213g tin wild red salmon with juice
115g/4oz self-raising flour
1 large organic egg
1 tbs olive oil
1 large tbs natural honey

Preheat oven to 190°C/375°F/Gas Mark 5. Grease a 24 x 21 x ¾ cm deep baking tray.

Combine and mash all the ingredients together in a large bowl until the mixture comes together to make a soft dough.

Spread dough evenly over the baking tray, and bake for 15 minutes. Remove from the oven, let cool in the tray. Cut into small bite-size squares.

Keep in an airtight glass container in fridge for up to three days, or freeze for up to one month.

Variation
Substitute salmon with the following: 2 x 120g tins sardines or 1 x 160g tin tuna in sunflower oil.

Prairie Woof Jacks

4 tbs light olive oil
3 large tbs local honey
230g/8oz oats
1 large apple, grated
2 handfuls ground natural nuts

Preheat oven to 190°C / 375°F / Gas Mark 5. Grease a 20 x 29cm baking tray.

Heat oil in a large pan for a couple of minutes and stir in the honey, then add oats, apple and nuts. Mix well to a soft dough.

Spread mixture 1 cm deep onto the tray, pressing down evenly with the back of a tablespoon. Bake for 20–25 minutes.

Remove from the oven and let cool in the tray. Cut into small bite size-squares.

Keep in an airtight container for up to five days, or freeze for up to one month.

Hedgerow Hip Bites for Dogs

230g/8oz organic self-raising flour
2 large organic eggs
4 good handfuls ripe autumn rose hips (remove pips)
2 tbs organic honey
2 tbs olive oil

Preheat oven to 190°C / 375°F / Gas Mark 5. Grease a 20 x 29cm baking tray.

Mix together all the ingredients in a large bowl to form soft dough. Spread mixture 1 cm deep on the baking tray. Bake for 25–30 minutes until just firm.

Remove from the oven and let cool. Cut into small bite-size squares. Keep in an airtight container for up to five days, or freeze for up to one month.

Variation
Substitute hips with 1 large grated eating apple or 1 banana or 2 handfuls of blackberries.

K9/Feline Nature's Own Hotpot

230g/8oz free-range turkey or chicken mince
1 medium grated carrot
1 handful French green beans (cut small)
1 handful basmati rice
1 medium potato diced
2 cabbage leaves shredded

Place all of the above in a large pan and add enough water to cover all ingredients. Bring to the boil, then gently simmer for 30 minutes until most of the liquid has been absorbed (top up pan with water if it starts to dry out). Allow to cool. Keep in fridge for up to three days, or freeze for up to one month.

Songbird Savoury Seedcake

String
Empty small plastic pots (284ml yogurt or cream pots do nicely)
1 block of lard
115g/4oz good-quality bird seed
115g/4oz raisins
115g/4oz natural peanuts
1 good handful of grated cheese

First, prepare your 'serving dishes'. For each plastic pot, take a piece of string about 20cm/9in long and thread through the base of the pot. Tie a knot at the end of the string and pull down about 2 inches to the inner edge of the pot. Allow yourself plenty of string at the other end to tie to a branch of a tree or bird stand.

Allow the lard to soften at room temperature. Cut up into pieces and place into a mixing bowl. Add the rest of the ingredients and mix together, then, using your hands, stuff the mixture into the pots. Make sure that you have enough string free. Place in the fridge to set hard.

When completely hard, take a knife and loosen away from the edge, pull off the plastic pot, then hang the seedcake outside.

Glossary of Herbs

This Glossary provides the common and Latin names for base oils, waters and macerated and essential oils mentioned in this book and that I keep on hand in my apothecary for natural healing.

Base Materials

Aloe vera (*Aloe barbadensis*) – the perfect topical base material, excellent used 'neat' or mixed with essential oils.

Olive oil (*Olea europaea*) – a gentle and versatile base oil.

Sunflower oil (*Helianthus annuus*)

Water – yes, plain old H_2O – is a very good medium for a range of healing plant materials.

Among the aromatic waters, I often have use for cornflower water (*Centaurea cyanus*).

Dried Herbs and Plant Material

Bladderwrack – *Fucus vesiculosus*

Borage – *Borago officinalis*

Catnip flowers – *Nepeta cataria*

Chickweed – *Stellaria media*

Clay

Devil's claw – *Harpagophytum procumberis*

Garlic – *Allium sativum*

Nettle/stinging nettle – *Urtica dioca*

Peppermint – *Mentha x piperita*

Rose hips – *Rosa canina*

Macerated Oils

Arnica (flowers) – *Arnica Montana*

Carrot – *Daucus carota ssp. sativus* or *D.Carota sp.carota*

Chickweed – *Stellaria media*

Comfrey – *Symphytum officinale*

Calendula – *Calendula officinalis*

Flaxseed or linseed – *Linum usitatissimum*

Hemp seed – *Cannabis sativa*

Neem – *Azadirachta indica*

St John's wort – *Hypericum perforatum*

Essential Oils

Angelica root – *Angelica archangelica*

Bay laurel – *Laurus nobilis*

Bergamot – *Citrus bergamia*

Carrot seed (wild) – *Daucus carota*

Chamomile, German – *Matricaria recutita*

Chamomile, Roman – *Anthemis nobilis* or *Chamaemelum nobile*

Citronella – *Cymbopogon nardus*

Clary sage – *Salvia sclarea*

Eucalyptus – *Eucalyptus radiata*

Garlic – *Allium sativum*

Lavender – *Lavendula officinalis* or *Lavandula angustifolia*

Lemon grass – *Cymbopogon citratus*

Nutmeg – *Myristica fragrans*

Orange blossom / neroli – *Citrus aurantium ssp. aurantium*

Peppermint – *Mentha* x *piperita*

Rose – *Rosa damascena*

Rosemary – *Rosmarinus officinalis*

Sandalwood – *Santalum album*

Seaweed absolute – *Fucus vesiculosus*

Tea tree – *Melaleuca alternifolia*

Thyme – *Thymus vulgaris*

Violet leaf, absolute – *Viola adorata*

Wintergreen – *Gaultheria procumbens*

Yarrow – *Achillea millefolium*

Further Reading
and Resources

Richard Allport, *Natural Healthcare for Pets* (Element Books, 2001)

Jack Angelo, *Your Healing Power* (Piatkus Books, 2007)

Jack and Jan Angelo, *Sacred Healing* (Piatkus Books, 2001)

Deepak Chopra, *How to Know God* (Rider & Co, 2001)

Nicholas Culpepper, *Culpeper's Complete Herbal* (many editions available)

------, *Culpeper's Colour Herbal* (Foulsham, 2006)

HH Dalai Lama, *The Art of Happiness* (Mobius, 1999)

Dr Wayne W. Dyer, *The Power of Intention* (Hay House, 2004)

Cindy Engel, *Wild Health* (Houghton Mifflin, 2003)

Louise L. Hay, *You Can Heal Your Life* (Hay House, 2004)

Caroline Ingraham, *The Animal Aromatics Workbook* (Caroline Ingraham, 2006)

Amelia Kinkade, *The Language of Miracles* (New World Library 2006)

Robert McDowell and Di Rowling, *Herbal Horsekeeping* (J A Allen & Co Ltd, 2003)

Kelly Marks, *Perfect Manners* (Ebury Press, 2002)

Cesar Millan, *Be the Pack Leader* (Hodder & Stoughton, 2008)

Penelope Ody, *Lifting the Spirit: Nature's Remedies for Stress and Relaxation* (Souvenir Press, 2003)

Dr Christine Page, *Frontiers of Health* (Rider & Co, 2005)

Kymythy R. Schulze, *Natural Nutrition for Dogs and Cats* (Hay House, 2003)

Hilary Page Self, *A Modern Horse Herbal* (Kenilworth Press, 2006)

Kim Sheridan, *Animals and the Afterlife* (Hay House, 2006)

Gordon Smith, *The Amazing Power of Animals* (Hay House, 2008)

Neale Donald Walsch, *Conversations with God* (Hodder Mobius, 1997)

Mary L. Wulff-Tilford and Gregory L. Tilford, *All You Ever Wanted to Know About Herbs for Pets* (BowTie Press, 1999)

Resources

Elizabeth Whiter
PO Box 25
HASSOCKS
BN6 8WN
www.elizabethwhiter.com
elizabeth@healinganimals.org

Elizabeth runs regular zoopharmacognosy and healing weekends as well as animal healing diploma courses. Email info@healinganimals.org for further details and booking forms.

Liz's animal healing diploma course is amazing. It combines the left and right brain in a perfect balance of anatomy and physiology, animal behaviour, meditation and communication. The practical work covered throughout the course enabled us to experience healing first-hand, and the case studies and dissertations demonstrated the

need to take our education and professionalism seriously.
The need to look after the animal owner or carer as well as the
animal was reinforced from the start, with learning human healing
and communication skills a fundamental part of the diploma.
All in all, this is a leap forward in developing a comprehensive,
professional workforce of animal healers who take their work
seriously and can therefore be taken seriously by clients and fellow
professionals alike. Oh, and did I say? – It is amazing fun, the
networking and friendships that we make are life-long!

Dr Alison Grimston MBBS BSc MPhil MRCGP MNFSH
Graduate of Animal Healing Diploma & Equine Diploma

To find a registered animal healer near you who has trained
in the diploma in animal and equine healing and workshops
with Elizabeth Whiter please visit:

www.healinganimals.org

Donkey and Horse Protection Charities
drupal.thedonkeysanctuary.org.uk
www.thebrooke.org
www.equinemarketwatch.org.uk

Celia Hammond Animal Trust
www.celiahammond.org

Cats Protection
www.cats.org.uk

Battersea Dogs & Cats Home
www.battersea.org.uk

Nicosia Dog Shelter
www.dogshelter.org.cy

Wildlife
www.specialistwildlifeservices.org

Royal Society for the Protection of Birds (RSPB)
www.rspb.org.uk

The Swan Sanctuary
www.swanuk.org.uk

The Parrot Society
www.theparrotsocietyuk.org

Bat Conservation Trust
http://www.bats.org.uk/

Fancy-Rats UK
www.fancy-rats.co.uk

Rabbit Welfare Association & Fund
www.rabbitwelfare.co.uk

Animal Rescuers
www.animalrescuers.co.uk

Compassion in World Farming
www.ciwf.org.uk

Animal Welfare Act
www.defra.gov.uk/animalh/welfare/act/index.htm

Paws Animal Sanctuary
www.pawsanimalsanctuaryfindon.co.uk

The Acorn Project
www.acornproject.co.uk

World Wildlife Fund
www.wwf.org.uk

Holistic Healthcare for Pets
www.thenaturallyhealthypet.com

Natural Therapies for Pets
www.TheNaturallyHealthyPet.com

National Federation of Spiritual Healers
www.nfsh.org.uk

Index

liver complaints 60

nervousness 21, 28, 51, 52, 72, 83, 108, 136
nettles 10, 11, 15, 32, 226
new surroundings 21, 29, 51, 161, 182

osteopathy xxii–xxiii, 206
overactive thyroid 28, 43

parasites 13, 34, 81, 94, 188
pregnancy 4

rescue dogs 15, 50, 102, 128, 159, 160–161
rose hips 10, 15, 153, 185, 190, 191, 195, 201, 222, 226
Royal College of Veterinary Surgeons 1, 189

self-esteem xviii, 54, 85, 101, 126, 175
separation 17, 182
skin irritations 34, 60, 79, 193
socialization 50, 160, 161
spiritual healing 1, 22, 99, 187
stiffening of joints 18, 65, 84, 128, 136, 192, 216
stomach tumours 60, 71, 76, 87, 92

ulcers 60

vertebrae damage xx, 78

worms 13

zoopharmacognosy xxv, 12, 13, 15, 20, 23, 25, 30, 59, 122, 187, 191

Notes

Notes

Notes

Notes

Notes

Notes

Notes

Notes

Notes

Notes

Notes

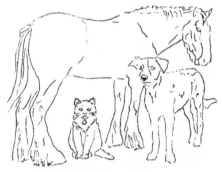

Diploma

in

Animal Healing

with

Elizabeth Whiter
MHAO MNFSH IIZ ITEC

1 year part-time courses

- ➢ Small Animals
- ➢ Equine

Enquiries:
elizabeth@healinganimals.org
www.healinganimals.org

JOIN THE HAY HOUSE FAMILY

As the leading self-help, mind, body and spirit publisher in the UK, we'd like to welcome you to our family so that you can enjoy all the benefits our website has to offer.

 EXTRACTS from a selection of your favourite author titles

 COMPETITIONS, PRIZES & SPECIAL OFFERS Win extracts, money off, downloads and so much more

 LISTEN to a range of radio interviews and our latest audio publications

 CELEBRATE YOUR BIRTHDAY An inspiring gift will be sent your way

 LATEST NEWS Keep up with the latest news from and about our Authors

 ATTEND OUR AUTHOR EVENTS Be the first to hear about our author events

 IPHONE APPS Download your favourite app for your iPhone

 HAY HOUSE INFORMATION Ask us anything, all enquiries answered

join us online at **www.hayhouse.co.uk**

 292B Kensal Road, London W10 5BE
T: 020 8962 1230 E: info@hayhouse.co.uk

We hope you enjoyed this Hay House book.
If you would like to receive a free catalogue featuring additional
Hay House books and products, or if you would like information
about the Hay Foundation, please contact:

Hay House UK Ltd
292B Kensal Road • London W10 5BE
Tel: (44) 20 8962 1230; Fax: (44) 20 8962 1239
www.hayhouse.co.uk

***

Published and distributed in the United States of America by:
Hay House, Inc. • PO Box 5100 • Carlsbad, CA 92018-5100
Tel: (1) 760 431 7695 or (1) 800 654 5126;
Fax: (1) 760 431 6948 or (1) 800 650 5115
www.hayhouse.com

***

Published and distributed in Australia by:
Hay House Australia Ltd • 18/36 Ralph Street • Alexandria, NSW 2015
Tel: (61) 2 9669 4299, Fax: (61) 2 9669 4144
www.hayhouse.com.au

***

Published and distributed in the Republic of South Africa by:
Hay House SA (Pty) Ltd • PO Box 990 • Witkoppen 2068
Tel/Fax: (27) 11 467 8904
www.hayhouse.co.za

***

Published and distributed in India by:
Hay House Publishers India • Muskaan Complex • Plot No.3
B-2 • Vasant Kunj • New Delhi - 110 070
Tel: (91) 11 41761620; Fax: (91) 11 41761630
www.hayhouse.co.in

***

Distributed in Canada by:
Raincoast • 9050 Shaughnessy St • Vancouver, BC V6P 6E5
Tel: (1) 604 323 7100
Fax: (1) 604 323 2600

***

Sign up via the Hay House UK website to receive the Hay House
online newsletter and stay informed about what's going on with your
favourite authors. You'll receive bimonthly announcements
about discounts and offers, special events, product highlights,
free excerpts, giveaways, and more!
www.hayhouse.co.uk